Sexual Health Matters in Primary Care

Gill Wakley

and

Ruth Chambers

Foreword by
Michael Adler

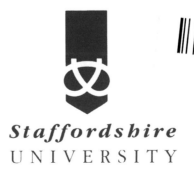

Staffordshire
UNIVERSITY

Radcliffe Medical Press Ltd
18 Marcham Road
Abingdon
Oxon OX14 1AA
United Kingdom

www.radcliffe-oxford.com
The Radcliffe Medical Press electronic catalogue and online ordering facility.
Direct sales to anywhere in the world.

British Library Cataloguing in Publication Data

A catalogue record for this book is available from the British Library.

ISBN 1 85775 414 X

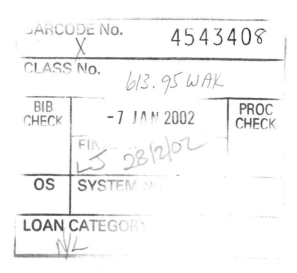
Typeset by Joshua Associates Ltd, Oxford
Printed and bound by TJ International Ltd, Padstow, Cornwall

Contents

Foreword

The recently published National Strategy for Sexual Health and HIV emphasised that 'sexual health is an important part of physical and mental health' and proposes a comprehensive and holistic model to deal with sexual health and HIV. Sexual health is a key part of our identity as human beings together with the fundamental human rights to privacy, a family life, and living free from discrimination. The central elements of good sexual health are equitable relationships and sexual fulfillment with access to information and services to avoid the risk of unintended pregnancy, illness or disease. The strategy recognises the very significant role that primary care teams can play in improving the nation's sexual health. It also recognises that everyone working in this field needs training. This will include people with a role in the delivery of HIV and STI prevention, education and services, and also people working with users, to help provide better sexual health services. Many disciplines will be involved, and all need to feel competent and empowered to deal with the issues around sexuality and sexual health.

In the light of the strategy, this book is important in its delivery. It outlines a comprehensive approach to the issues of sexual health, touching on the working environment, especially creating an atmosphere within practices which allows ease of access and reduction of the inevitable stigma that tends to go with these issues. It also gives basic approaches to best practice and the clinical management of sexual health matters. In view of the increasing importance of primary care in providing sexual health services, this is an invaluable book which will form the basis for any general practice team wishing to do better.

Michael Adler
Professor of Genitourinary Medicine
Department of Sexually Transmitted Diseases
Royal Free & University College Medical School
September 2001

About the authors

Gill Wakley started in general practice in 1966, but transferred to community medicine shortly afterwards and then into public health. A desire for increased contact with patients caused her to move back into general practice, together with community gynaecology, in 1978. She has been combining the two, in varying amounts, ever since. Throughout she has been heavily involved in learning and teaching. She was in a training general practice, and became a Member of the Faculty of Family Planning and Reproductive Health Care (RCOG) and a Member of the Institute of Psychosexual Medicine. She was until recently a Senior Clinical Lecturer with the Primary Care Department at Keele University, Staffordshire. Like Ruth, she has run all types of educational initiatives and activities, from individual mentoring and instruction to small group work, plenary lectures, distance-learning programmes, workshops, and courses for a wide range of health professionals and lay people. She obtained an MD (Keele University) for her investigation into the provision for sexual health in primary care.

Ruth Chambers has been a GP for more than 20 years and is currently the Professor of Primary Care Development at Staffordshire University. She has undertaken a wide range of research and development focusing on stress and the health of doctors, health at work and the quality of healthcare. Ruth has designed and organised many types of educational initiatives, including distance-learning programmes. Recently she has developed a keen interest in working with GPs, nurses and others in primary care around clinical governance and practice personal and professional development plans. She is currently leading a national project to identify innovative educational tools that will help to reduce teenage pregnancy rates.

Glossary of common abbreviations and terms used

AIDS	Autoimmune deficiency syndrome
Case–control study	Each person in the study is matched (usually by at least age and sex) to one or more other individuals who are not exposed to the substance, illness or intervention being researched
COC	Combined oral contraceptive
Cohort study	A group of people being studied is matched to a group that is not being exposed to that risk or suffering from the condition being studied
Critical incident analysis	The systematic analysis of a particular incident to establish beneficial or adverse effects on the outcome[1]
DFFP	Diploma of the Faculty of Family Planning (of the Royal College of Obstetricians and Gynaecologists)
GP	General practitioner
Guidelines	A written account of how a condition or intervention might be managed in the best way, customary way or to minimum standards
HIV	Human immunodeficiency virus
HPV	Human papilloma virus
Incidence	The frequency of first or new episodes of a condition in a defined population
IUD; IUCD	Intrauterine device; intrauterine contraceptive device
Meta-analysis	A statistical procedure designed to combine the results of several studies, but which cannot correct for variations in the quality or methodology of the original studies

MFFP	Membership of the Faculty of Family Planning (of the Royal College of Obstetricians and Gynaecologists)
NSF	National Service Framework – the standards published by the Department of Health for the management of certain priority conditions
Observational studies	Studies that look for associations between disease and exposure to known or suspected risk factors, or between interventions and progress of the disease
PCO	Primary care organisation – includes both primary care trusts and primary care groups, local health groups in Wales, local health co-operatives in Scotland, and health and social care groups in Northern Ireland
PDP	Personal development plan
Placebo	An inactive intervention or substance used in a trial
POP	Progestogen-only pill
PPDP	Practice or workplace personal and professional development plan
Prevalence	In a defined population, the rate of all cases of a condition, whether they are new or continuing
Protocol	A written set of rules for the management of a condition or for an intervention
RCT	Randomised controlled trial – two comparison groups selected by chance alone are used, one of which receives the intervention while the other receives no intervention, a comparison intervention or a placebo
Relative risk (RR)	One risk is given the score of unity (1) and other risks are compared with it; the ratio between the disease rate in individuals who are exposed to a risk factor and those who are not exposed to it
Shared care	An arrangement whereby the management of a patient's condition is shared between health professionals from different disciplines or organisations
SIGN	Scottish Intercollegiate Guidelines Network
Significant event auditing	An audit of an incident to establish beneficial or adverse effects and then make changes (if required)

Single group pre–post testing	A single group that has indicators required for the study recorded before and after exposure to the substance or intervention
STI	Sexually transmitted infection
Systematic review	An academic research approach to reviewing the literature on a particular subject using guidelines to collect and grade all of the evidence on the subject[2]
Time series	An approach that involves using a small group of people and following them up carefully over (usually) long periods of time to determine the outcome and modifying factors

References

1 Clarke R and Croft P (1998) *Critical Reading for the Reflective Practitioner*. Reed Educational & Professional Publishing, Butterworth-Heinemann, Oxford.
2 Chalmers I and Altman DG (1995) *Systematic Reviews*. BMJ Publishing Group, London.

Introduction

The material in this book sets out how learning more about sexual health matters and reviewing current practice can be incorporated into the personal development plans of large numbers of people. These include GPs, practice nurses, reception staff and practice managers, as well as community family planning nurses and doctors, midwives and health visitors, school nurses and district nurses, therapists, pharmacists and supporting clerical and administrative staff. Many individuals working in other settings will also find it useful, such as doctors, nurses and health advisers in genitourinary clinics, health staff in gynaecology and rheumatology departments, and those who encounter people and their sexual health problems in various health and social care disciplines. There is a dual focus on best practice in the clinical management of sexual health matters and improving the working environment so that the practice or workplace systems and procedures are well organised. Practice and workplace teams should work together to direct their individual learning plans to form their practice or workplace personal and professional development plan, which complements the business plan of the practice, workplace or primary care organisation. Primary care organisations in the UK include primary care groups and trusts, local health groups in Wales, the local healthcare co-operatives in Scotland or the primary care co-operatives in Northern Ireland. The principles described apply to any health staff or groups of health professionals and managers who are trying to improve the quality of care for their patients who have sexual health needs.

This programme is focused on sexual health matters because of their importance as described in the introduction to the consultation for the sexual health strategy by the Department of Health for England (*see* list of website addresses in the Appendix). This states that:

'The sexual health of the nation is of great concern to the Government. There are a number of indicators of poor sexual health.

- In 1997 the conception rate for girls under the age of 16 years was 8.9 per 1000. For girls aged 15–19 years, the rate was 62.3 per 1000. These are the highest rates of teenage pregnancies in Western Europe. There is wide variation across the country and there are also wide variations within health authority areas.

- Half of all conceptions in under-16-year-olds and more than one-third of conceptions in 16 to 19-year-olds end in an abortion. There was a rise in the number of abortions in all age groups in 1998. Abortions rose by 11% in those under 20 years of age and by 6% in those over 30 years of age.
- Even though considerable publicity has been given to teenagers, it is important to remember that 80% (130 000) of the total number of terminations of pregnancy per year occur in women beyond their teenage years.
- The incidence of virtually all sexually transmitted infections (STIs) is increasing. The number of attendances at departments of genito-urinary medicine for sexually transmitted infections now totals 1 million per year, representing a doubling over the last decade. The commonest conditions are genital warts (associated with the sub-sequent development of carcinoma of the cervix), chlamydia and gonorrhoea (which if untreated can result in ectopic pregnancy and infertility). The number of cases of chlamydial infection seen in genitourinary clinics has risen by 21% between 1996 and 1997, and by a further 13% between 1997 and 1998 (*see* Chapter 6). Population surveys have reported rates of chlamydia infection as high as 25%, particularly in young women.
- There has been no reduction in the annual number of new diagnoses of HIV made, and the latest annual figures saw the highest number of new HIV diagnoses ever recorded (*see* Chapter 7).'

There are likely to be changes in the way in which sexual health services are provided (*see* Box 1) following the publication of the sexual health strategy. It is envisaged that much more sexual healthcare and promotion will take place in primary care. Every primary care team, together with community genitourinary and family planning services, community pharmacists and youth services, should be able to:

- take a sexual history and assess sexual risk taking
- provide oral contraception and give information about the full range of contraceptive options, as well as where to obtain them
- provide pregnancy testing and appropriate referral
- provide cervical cytology testing and referral
- test symptomatic women for STIs
- assess and refer men with symptoms of STIs
- provide hepatitis B screening and immunisation
- provide HIV counselling and referral.

Box 1 Possible scheme for provision of sexual health services

Patient and partner(s) attend by:

Self-referral at primary care level	• Primary care team in general practices • Community contraceptive and sexual health clinics • Genitourinary clinics with links to other services, such as schools, youth organisations, outreach workers, etc., in the community
Referral by health professional, or self-referral at intermediate level	• General practitioners and nurses with a special interest and qualifications • Outreach services provided by community contraceptive care, genitourinary clinics, gynaecology, etc.
Referral by health professional at secondary care level	• Specialist services in secondary care

---

In addition, specialised generalist services could support general practitioners who have a special interest in providing specialist-interest primary care teams, perhaps for the primary care organisation (PCO) or for several PCOs. They might include genitourinary specialist provision and community contraceptive services.[1] Other services that this level of provision might include would be STI testing for men, partner tracing and notification, long-acting contraception, management of psychosexual problems, and vasectomy.

All of these services will need to interface with more specialist services. Termination of pregnancy could take place in secondary care, although more local community provision at primary or inter-mediate level is being piloted in various areas.[2,3] Specialist STI manage-ment and specialist HIV management and care should be undertaken in secondary care. Gynaecological management of some complex dis-orders (e.g. pelvic inflammatory disease, vulval disease, intrauterine device complications, etc.) also requires referral to secondary care.

Female sterilisation has usually been a secondary care activity, but again can be performed without general anaesthesia in selected patients in community settings.

Learning needs will arise from the increased role of primary care in the management of straightforward sexual health matters, and the role of doctors and nurses with a special interest in sexual health at intermediate level. These relate not only to those individuals who are involved in direct clinical care, but also to those who are providing the resources and services for these activities to take place in a well-provisioned and well-run manner.

You may decide to allocate 50% of the time you intend to spend on drawing up, justifying and applying a personal development plan in any one year to best practice in sexual health matters. That would leave space in your learning plan for other important topics, such as mental health, coronary heart disease or cancer – whatever is a priority for you, your post and your patient population.

The first chapter of the book describes how a clinical governance culture incorporates good clinical management as well as good service provision that is accessible and equitable. You should be able to demonstrate that you are fit to practise as an individual clinician or manager (best practice in the management of sexual health matters), and that your working environment is fit to practise from (a well-organised practice or workplace). This section will be relevant to all readers, whether you are a clinician, an employee or a manager, so that you understand more of the context within which you work and how your individual contribution fits into the whole picture of healthcare.

The chapters that follow provide important information about the management of some of the more common, or more serious, sexual health conditions, together with references so that you can find out more about particular subjects. To make it easier to retrieve information, references are usually made to reviews or summaries rather than to a large number of original documents. Many changes in clinical management have occurred in recent years – for example, in the treatment of impotence or in recognising the importance of identifying infections with chlamydia. Many of the clinical or service areas could be the subject of a personal development plan in their own right. Decide how wide or narrow your own focus will be and select what is manageable within a reasonable time-scale, rather than trying to cover everything in one year.

The material in the chapters that follow is designed to help to point you in the right direction in your search for information about sexual health matters. The whole programme builds up to help you to generate a personal development plan in Chapter 10, or a practice or workplace personal and professional development plan in Chapter 11. Interactive exercises at the end of each chapter give you an opportunity to undertake an assessment of your learning needs, review your own performance or the efficiency of your practice or workplace organisation, and reflect on what improvements you could make.

You should transfer information from these needs assessment exercises to the relevant slots in the personal development plan if you are following this programme as an individual, or the practice or workplace personal and professional development plan if you are working as a team. Adopt a wide-based approach to improving quality – think of how you are establishing a clinical governance culture in your own practice or workplace team in your timed action plans.

What should you do next?

Study the blank template for a personal development plan on pages 148–158, or for a practice or workplace personal and professional development plan on pages 174–181. You will be filling one of these in as you go along. Decide whether you will be starting out on your personal development plan or working with colleagues on the practice or workplace learning plan. You will need to ensure that everyone's personal development plans mesh with the practice or workplace learning plan by the end.[4,5]

Make changes as a result – to your workplace, or to the equipment and its use, or to the advice you give to patients, or the way in which you manage and investigate sexual health matters or organise their prevention. Build in ways in which you can evaluate how well the changes have worked.

References

1 Wilkinson C (2000) The integration of family planning and genitourinary services. *Br J Fam Plan Reprod Health Care.* **26**: 187–9.
2 Boorer C and Murty J (2001) Experiences of termination of pregnancy in a stand-alone clinic situation. *Br J Fam Plan Reprod Health Care.* **27**: 97–8.
3 Wilson S (2001) Meeting the need for induced abortion. *Br J Fam Plan Reprod Health Care.* **27**: 93–6.

4 Chambers R and Wakley G (2000) *Making Clinical Governance Work for You.* Radcliffe Medical Press, Oxford.

5 Wakley G, Chambers R and Field S (2000) *Continuing Professional Development in Primary Care: making it happen.* Radcliffe Medical Press, Oxford.

CHAPTER 1

Clinical governance and the management of sexual health matters

Introduction

The range of sexual health matters is very wide, and overlaps occur between the specialties of contraception, gynaecology and genitourinary medicine, as well as between other disciplines involved in the care of patients with these conditions. Many patients do not regard themselves as 'ill' but rather as suffering from 'dis-ease' in the wider sense of the word (or from potential harm, such as an unwanted pregnancy), and consideration of their social and psychological well-being plays a significant part in their management. A selection of topics has been made to represent what might be of concern to a healthcare team that is aiming to improve the management of this particular part of their workload.

Sexual health has been defined as 'Enjoyment of the sexual activity of one's choice, without causing or experiencing physical or emotional harm'.[1]

Clinical governance is inclusive, making quality everyone's business, whether they are a doctor, a nurse, a pharmacist or other independent contractor, a manager, a member of staff or a strategic planner. We need to know where we are now, and where we want to get to, if we are to drive up standards of healthcare.

Clinical governance has been defined as doing 'anything and everything required to maximise quality'.[2,3] Clinical governance should create a culture and working environment in which people thrive and feel fulfilled by their work but where, at the same time, under-performance is identified and corrected.

Components of clinical governance

The components of clinical governance are not new. However, bringing them together under the banner of clinical governance and introducing more explicit accountability for performance is a new style of working.

The following 14 themes are core components of professional and service development which together form a comprehensive approach to providing high-quality healthcare services and clinical governance.[3] These are illustrated in Figure 1.1.

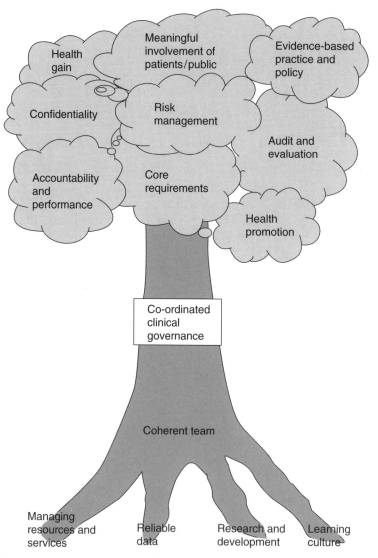

Figure 1.1: 'Routes' and branches of clinical governance.

If you interweave these 14 components into your individual and workplace-based personal and professional development plans you will have addressed the requirements for clinical governance at the same time.[4]

1   *Learning culture*: in the practice or workplace, primary care organisation or department.
2   *Research and development culture*: in the practice or workplace, or throughout the health service.
3   *Reliable and accurate data*: in the practice or workplace, or across the NHS as a seamless whole.
4   *Well-managed resources and services*: as individuals, as a practice or workplace, across the NHS and in conjunction with other organisations.
5   *Coherent team*: well-integrated teams within a practice or workplace, including attached staff.
6   *Meaningful involvement of patients and the public*: including users, carers and the general population.
7   *Health gain*: activities to improve the health of staff and patients in a practice or workplace, a primary care organisation or a department.
8   *Confidentiality*: of information in consultations, in medical notes, and between healthcare staff.
9   *Evidence-based practice and policy*: applying it in practice or in the workplace, in the district, and across the NHS.
10 *Accountability and performance*: for standards, performance of individuals, the practice or the workplace, both to the public and to those in authority.
11 *Core requirements*: good fit with skill mix and whether individuals are competent to do their jobs; communication, work-force numbers, and morale at practice or workplace level.
12 *Health promotion*: for patients, the public, your staff and colleagues – both opportunistic and in general, or targeting those with most needs.
13 *Audit and evaluation*: for instance, of the extent to which individuals and practice or workplace teams adhere to best practice in clinical management or human resources.
14 *Risk management*: being competent to detect those at risk, and reducing the risks and probabilities of ill health.

The challenges to delivering clinical governance

Delivering high-quality healthcare with guaranteed minimum standards of care for users at all times is a major challenge. At present, the quality of healthcare is patchy and variable. We are not very good at detecting under-performance and then taking the initiative and rectifying it at an early stage. The small number of clinicians who do under-perform exert a disproportionately large effect on the public's confidence. Causes of under-performance in an individual might be a result of a lack of knowledge or skills, poor attitudes or ill health. There is too much variation in the provision available to patients.

Box 1.1

In one area there may be a variety of places where people can obtain emergency contraception, including several general practice surgeries (whether the women are registered there or not), open-access contraceptive and sexual health clinics, NHS Direct drop-in surgeries, pharmacies, and even the Accident and Emergency centre. In another area emergency contraception may only be available if the woman travels to a clinic some distance away, assuming that she can be fitted in after a long wait at an appointment-only facility.

However, a lack of management capability is nearly always an important factor contributing to inadequate clinical services, and provision can be patchy.

Box 1.2

Facilities for taking swabs to identify vaginal infections may be standard in one area but very limited in others, due to lack of time and financial resources, or because of difficulties in transporting specimens in good condition within a reasonable time period.

We need to understand why variation exists and explore ways of reducing inequalities. Variation in the quality of healthcare provided is common – between different practices or units in the same locality, between staff of the same discipline working in the same practice or unit, and between care given to some groups of the population rather than others.

Clinical governance offers a co-ordinated approach to overcoming these areas of risk through a combination of clinical and organisational improvements to the quality of healthcare practice.

Learning culture

Education and training programmes should be relevant to service needs, whether at organisational or individual levels. Continuing professional development (CPD) programmes need to meet both the learning needs of individual health professionals and the wider service development needs of the NHS. You should no longer opt for CPD activities according to what you *want* to do, but rather according to what you *need* to do. Clinical governance underpins professional and service development.

Box 1.3

Individual personal development plans
will feed into a
workplace or practice-based personal and professional development plan
that will feed into
the organisation's business plan,
all of which are
underpinned by clinical governance.[4]

Therefore focusing on sexual health matters would be a good topic for a practice or workplace personal and professional development plan with a mix of learning about the effective clinical management of sexual health matters in an efficient work environment.

Applying research and development in practice

The conclusions of the many thousands of research papers about sexual health matters that are published in reputable journals each year are rarely applied in practice. This is because few health professionals or managers make time to read such journals systematically, and therefore they are unaware of the research findings. Furthermore, most practice or workplace teams do not have a system for reviewing important research papers and translating that review into practical action. The primary care organisation might help by feeding important new evidence to its constituent practices and workplaces, as well as to pharmacies, clinics or indeed the general public, with suggestions or templates for making changes in practice, backed by resources to enable change to happen. The incorporation of research-based evidence into everyday practice should promote policies on effective working and improve quality and a clinical governance culture.

Box 1.4

There is evidence that the detection and prompt treatment of chlamydial infection, together with contact tracing of sexual partners, can reduce the subsequent risk of pelvic inflammatory disease, tubal infertility and ectopic pregnancy.[5] Surveys of the management of chlamydial infection have shown that there is room for considerable improvement in the way in which chlamydia is detected, treated and followed up.[6]

Reliable and accurate data

Clinicians, patients and administrators need reliable and accurate data to connect individuals or their healthcare records to other knowledge that is relevant to the care of the patient. Set the following standards for workplaces.

- Keep records in chronological order.
- Summarise medical records, within a specified time period for records of new patients.
- Review dates for checks on medication, with audit in place to monitor adherence to standards and plan what to do in the event of under-performance if necessary.
- Use computers for diagnostic recording.
- Record information from external sources (e.g. hospital, other organisations) that is relevant to individual patients or the workplace.

Keep good written records of policies and audits that relate to sexual health matters in the practice or workplace. An inspection at any time should show what audits have been undertaken and when, the changes in practice or workplace organisation that followed, the extent of staff training undertaken, and the future programme of monitoring.

Well-managed resources and services

The things you need to achieve best practice should be in the right place at the right time and working correctly every time.

Set standards in your practice or workplace for the following:

- access to premises and availability of services for people with special needs (e.g. those with disability)
- provision of routine and urgent appointments
- access to and provision for referral for investigation or treatment
- pro-active monitoring of chronic illness and disability
- alternatives to face-to-face consultations
- consultation length.

The six primary care services to which the public requires access are information, advice, triage and treatment, continuity of care, personal care and other services.[7]

Systems should be designed to prevent and detect errors. Therefore keep systems simple and sensible, and inform everyone how those systems operate so that they are less likely to bypass the system or make errors. This certainly applies to follow-up of patients' clinical management.

Coherent teamwork

Teams produce better patient care than single practitioners can when operating in a fragmented way. Effective teams make the most of the different contributions of individual clinical disciplines in delivering patient care. The characteristics of effective teams are as follows:

- shared ownership of a common purpose
- clear goals for the contributions that each discipline makes
- open communication between team members
- opportunities for team members to enhance their skills.

A team approach helps different team members to adopt an evidence-based approach to patient care – by having to justify their approach to the rest of the team.[8]   Sexual health matters are conditions that require teamwork in order to achieve the best results for individual patients. The primary care team may include GPs and practice nurses, non-clinical staff and community pharmacists, youth and community services, school nurses and educational services, and often extends to include shared care with secondary care services.

Meaningful involvement of patients and the public

People use terms like 'user' or 'consumer' to describe who we should be involving in giving us feedback about the quality or type of healthcare that we offer, or in planning future services. Patients or carers, non-users of services, the local community, a particular subgroup of the population or the general public will all have useful feedback and views. For example, they might provide information on the accessibility of your own practice or workplace premises, or your systems that inform people about the results of investigations or queries.

If user involvement and public participation are effective, they should result in the following:

- reductions in health inequalities
- better outcomes of individual care
- better health of the population
- better quality and more locally responsive services
- greater ownership of health services
- a better understanding of why and how local services need to be changed and developed.

A meaningful public consultation involves the exchange of information between the healthcare providers and the general public, and obtaining a representative opinion as a result, that feeds into the local decision-making process of healthcare services or whoever is sponsoring the consultation.

Box 1.5

- You might want to consult the public and health professionals about the availability of emergency contraception or long-acting methods of contraception.
- You could select a group of representative patients to help to draw up innovative interventions to reduce the number of unwanted pregnancies or sexually transmitted infections in your area.

- You could target groups that are more difficult to reach, such as teenagers, men under 50 years of age, people with disabilities, or other specific groups who attend for healthcare less often than others.

It may be difficult or expensive to obtain representative opinions. You may have to trade off a relatively cheap method of consultation that engages with fewer people or with a less representative section of the population subgroup. If you do, you will need to understand what biases are arising and make allowances for those biases when you interpret the results of the consultation.[9]

Health gain

The two general approaches to improving health are the 'population' approach, which focuses on measures to improve health through the community, and the 'high-risk' approach, which focuses on vulnerable individuals who are at high risk of the condition or hazard.

The two approaches are not mutually exclusive, and they often need to be combined with legislation and community action. Health goals include:

- a good quality of life
- avoiding premature death
- equal opportunities for health.

Modifiable risk factors for reducing the adverse effects of sexual health matters include:

- postponement of early sexual activity
- safer sexual practices
- effective contact tracing and treatment of individuals with sexually transmitted infections.

Confidentiality

Confidentiality is a component of clinical governance that is often overlooked. Experienced health professionals and managers may assume that junior or new staff know all about confidentiality, when in fact they may not. There are many difficult situations in the workplace where one person asks for information about another individual's medical condition (e.g. test results or a progress report), where it is not clear-cut as to whether this information should be supplied or withheld. Sometimes it is not even clear whether the person being asked should acknowledge that the person being enquired about is under their care.

Box 1.6

Mr W telephones to ask for his wife's test results. He says that she is working and cannot ring herself during the day, so she has asked him to telephone. He becomes angry and demanding when the receptionist explains that she cannot tell him whether or not his wife has had any test results. Later the receptionist feels very relieved that she did adhere to the rules. When she passes on her account to the practice nurse (who would normally give the result to Mrs W), she hears that Mr and Mrs W are in the middle of an acrimonious divorce.

The Caldicott Committee Report describes the following principles of good practice to safeguard confidentiality when information is being used for non-clinical purposes.[10]

- Justify the purpose.
- Do not use patient-identifiable information unless it is absolutely necessary to do so.
- Use the minimum necessary patient-identifiable information.
- Access to patient-identifiable information should be on a strict need-to-know basis.
- Everyone with access to patient-identifiable information should be aware of his or her responsibilities.

Evidence-based culture

The key features that determined whether or not local guidelines worked in one initiative[11] were as follows.

- There was multidisciplinary involvement in drawing them up.
- A well-described systematic review of the literature underpinned the guidelines, with graded recommendations for best practice linked to the evidence.
- Ownership was nurtured at both national and local levels.

- A local implementation plan ensured that all of the practicalities (e.g. time, staff, education and training resources) were foreseen and met, stakeholders were supported, and predictors of sustainability were addressed (e.g. guideline usability, individualising guidelines to practitioners and patients).

Box 1.7

Guidelines on the management of genital chlamydial infection have been drawn up by the Scottish Intercollegiate Guidelines Network (SIGN) (publication number 42; *see* list of useful websites in Appendix) and list the grades of evidence on which they are based. SIGN publishes the grades that they use on the website, but the classification is under review. You may want to look at the paper referred to previously on evidence-based guidelines for the management of genital chlamydial infection to see how the Leicestershire Chlamydia Guidelines Group drew up their guidelines.[6]

There are several systems for grading evidence. One classification that is often quoted gives the strength of evidence as shown in Box 1.8.[12]

Box 1.8 Strength of evidence

Type I	Strong evidence from at least one systematic review of multiple well-designed randomised controlled trials (RCTs)
Type II	Strong evidence from at least one properly designed randomised controlled trial of appropriate size
Type III	Evidence from well-designed trials without randomisation, single group pre–post, cohort, time-series or matched case–control studies
Type IV	Evidence from well-designed non-experimental studies from more than one centre or research group
Type V	Opinions of respected authorities, based on clinical evidence, descriptive studies or reports of expert committees

---

This hierarchy of evidence is sometimes simplified into an ABC format (*see* SIGN website) as follows.

- A – required: at least one randomised controlled trial as part of the body of literature of overall good quality and consistency addressing specific recommendations.
- B – required: availability of well-conducted clinical studies but no randomised controlled trials on the topic of recommendation.
- C – required: evidence obtained from expert committee reports or opinions and/or clinical experience of respected authorities; indicates the absence of directly applicable clinical studies of good quality.

Other categories of evidence are listed in the compendium of the best available evidence for effective healthcare – *Clinical Evidence* – which is updated every six months, and is perhaps more useful to the health professional in everyday work (*see* Box 1.9).[13]

Box 1.9

Beneficial	Interventions whose effectiveness has been shown by clear evidence from controlled trials
Likely to be beneficial	Interventions for which effectiveness is less well established than for those listed under 'beneficial'
Trade-off between benefits and harms	Interventions for which clinicians and patients should weigh up the beneficial and harmful effects according to individual circumstances and priorities
Unknown effectiveness	Interventions for which there are currently insufficient data, or data of inadequate quality (this includes interventions that are widely accepted as beneficial but which have never been formally tested in RCTs, often because the latter would be regarded as unethical)
Unlikely to be beneficial	Interventions for which lack of effectiveness is less well established than for those listed under 'likely to be ineffective or harmful'
Likely to be ineffective or harmful	Interventions whose ineffectiveness or harmfulness has been demonstrated by clear evidence.

Accountability and performance

Health professionals may not always realise that they are accountable to others from outside their own professions, especially if they are of self-employed status, as are GPs and pharmacists. However, in fact they are accountable to:

- the general public, which is entitled to expect high standards of healthcare
- the profession – to maintain the standards of knowledge and skills of the profession as a whole
- the Government – and employer – who expect high standards of healthcare from the work-force.

Box 1.10

Health professionals who believe that they are not accountable to others may be reluctant to collect the evidence to demonstrate that they are fit to practise, and that their working environment is fit to practise from. They may be reluctant to co-operate with central NHS requirements, such as working to the National Service Frameworks or following Health Strategy plans.

Identify and rectify under-performance at an early stage by means of the following:

- regular appraisals (at least annually) linked to clinical governance and personal development plans. Appraisal is a process of regular meetings between manager and staff member, or between doctor or pharmacist and external appraiser or educational tutor, with support for the benefit of the person who is being appraised
- detecting those who have significant health problems, and referring them for help
- systematic audit that detects individuals' performance, as opposed to the overall performance of the practice or workplace team
- an open learning culture in which team members are discouraged from covering up colleagues' inadequacies, so that problems can be resolved at an early stage.

Clinicians may regard the performance assessment framework as a management tool that is not particularly relevant to their clinical practice. However, it does reinforce a clinical governance culture whereby good clinical management and organisational management have a symbiotic relationship.

> **Box 1.11**
>
> The NHS performance assessment framework has six components, namely health improvement, fair access, efficiency, effective delivery of appropriate care, user/carer experience and health outcomes.

Health promotion

People may underestimate relative risks as applied to themselves and their own behaviour. For example, many people accept the relationship between sexual intercourse and sexually transmitted infections, but do not believe that they personally are at risk. People usually have a reasonable idea of the *relative risks* of various activities and behaviours, although their personal estimates of the *magnitude* of those risks tend to be biased, with small probabilities often being over-estimated, and high probabilities often being under-estimated.

> **Box 1.12**
>
> At the height of the publicity about HIV and AIDS, many women changed their contraceptive method from oral contraceptives to condoms to improve their protection against the infection, but did not realise that by doing this they were reducing their protection against the greater risk of pregnancy.[14,15]

Audit and evaluation

Audit will probably be the method you think of first for determining what your needs are – as a clinician or as a practice or workplace. You might look at the extent to which you are adhering to practice, workplace or pharmacy protocols – for instance, whether you are consistently advising those who attend for emergency contraception about more reliable methods, or comparing other aspects of clinical care with best practice or workplace guidelines.

> **Box 1.13**
>
> It is recommended that you should record the blood pressure of all women before starting them on oral contraceptives, and that you should check it regularly thereafter.[16] You could set standards (e.g. 100% of women have their blood pressure measured before combined oral contraceptives are prescribed, and 90% of those on combined oral contraception have a recorded blood pressure level in the last 12 months). Then audit your records for compliance and take action before re-auditing if your results are not satisfactory.

Analysis of critical or significant incidents should focus on organisational factors, not just on the performance of particular individuals.

> **Box 1.14**
>
> A woman attends a GP surgery after the session for emergencies on a Saturday morning has finished and the doctor is out on visits. The receptionist gives her an appointment for Monday morning, as she says she 'needs the pill urgently'. On Monday, it is discovered that she wanted emergency contraception and is now outside the 72-hour time limit for oral methods. She is angry and upset that she now needs to return to see another doctor for an intrauterine device to be fitted instead. A review (significant event audit) of the circumstances prompts some changes. The receptionists learn more about contraception and receive some role-play training in dealing with potentially embarrassing situations at the reception desk. The practice nurses receive some extra training and take over more of the emergency contraception provision, and their hours are changed slightly so that there is better cover on Saturday mornings. No changes to the arrangements for intrauterine device fitting are made, as the number fitted in the practice does not justify this.

Core requirements

You cannot deliver clinical governance without well-trained and competent staff, the right skill mix of staff, and a safe and comfortable working environment that is providing cost-effective care. Following published referral guidelines may increase healthcare costs – which should be justifiable as cost-effective care when all direct and indirect costs are taken into account.

Your healthcare team can do much under the umbrella of clinical governance to respond to the government challenges to improve the following:

- *partnership*: working together across the NHS to ensure the best possible care
- *performance*: acting to review and deliver higher standards of healthcare
- *the professions and wider work-force*: breaking down barriers between different disciplines (e.g. through multidisciplinary team-work between GPs, nurses, pharmacists, school nurses and general practices)
- *patient care*: access, convenient services, and empowerment to take a full part in decision making about their own medical care and in planning and providing health services in general
- *prevention*: promoting healthy living across all sections of society and tackling variations in care.

Risk management

Risk management in general practice mainly centres on assessing probabilities that potential or actual hazards will give rise to harm. Consider how bad the risk is, how likely the risk is, when the risk will occur (if ever), and how certain you are of estimates about the risks. This applies just as much whether the risk is an environmental or organisational risk within the practice or workplace, or a clinical risk.

Box 1.15

While a GP is seeing a female patient for another condition, she asks if he will give her a Depo-Provera injection for her contraception, as the practice nurse is off sick. He goes into the treatment room and rummages around to find them, as he does not normally do this himself. He gives the patient the injection and then to his horror realises that he has just given Depo-Medrone instead. He apologises and goes back to find that the correct injection is stacked neatly next to the Depo-Medrone. The following day, after discussing this incident with his colleagues and the practice manager, the injections are placed in different cupboards and the doors of the cupboards are labelled appropriately. The GP resolves that in future he will record the batch number in the patient record *before* giving the injection, so that he has to examine it more closely beforehand.

Good practice means understanding and managing risk – both clinical and organisational aspects. Undertaking audit more systematically will reduce the risks of omission – both in detection and in clinical management. The common areas of risk in providing healthcare services are thought to include the following:[17]

- out-of-date clinical practice
- lack of continuity of care
- poor communication
- mistakes in patient care
- patient complaints
- financial risk – insufficient resources
- reputation
- staff morale.

Communicating and managing risks with regard to individual patients depends very much on finding ways to explain risks and elicit people's values and preferences so that all of these dimensions can be incorporated into the decisions they themselves make to take risks or to choose between alternatives that involve different risks and benefits. A well-functioning system through which patients can make complaints and receive feedback on the outcome should allow the practice or unit to reduce risks of a recurrence.

Box 1.16

A patient had asked for a prescription for an emergency packet of her usual contraceptive pill as she had left it too late to get an appointment in time to restart. She complained that she had been put at risk because she had been prescribed a pill that she had previously discontinued, not the one she was using currently. A significant incident analysis showed that the use of the new pill had not been recorded in her computerised medication record because it had been prescribed by hand on a day when the computer system was out of action. The procedure for adding manual records to the computer under these circumstances was reviewed and modified as a result, and the patient was mollified by being thanked for her input.

Reflection exercise

Exercise 1

Review and plan to improve your knowledge, attitudes and skills about sexual health matters.

Think how you might integrate the 14 components of clinical governance into your personal development plan. Examples are given for each component listed below. Try to complete this from your own perspective.

- *Establishing a learning culture*: e.g. arrange a session to update staff at a multidisciplinary meeting about guidelines and up-to-date information on the management of sexual health matters. Leave a folder containing 'interesting articles on sex' on the table in the common-room so that people can browse and keep up to date.
- *Managing resources and services*: e.g. inform primary care organisations or the unit management about shortfalls in laboratory services for identification of STIs, or the poor availability of secondary care facilities for termination of pregnancy. Arrange for nurse-run group protocols for emergency and continuing contraception.
- *Establishing a research and development culture*: e.g. undertake some research into sexual health matters, perhaps by linking with the local university or a research network. Share published papers citing evidence on sexual health matters with work colleagues when they might be of relevance to your patient management.
- *Reliable and accurate data*: e.g. record sexual health matters in a clear and consistent way so that you can repeat the exercise next year and compare the results.
- *Evidence-based practice and policy*: e.g. formulate a protocol for prescribing or referring for sexual health matters.
- *Confidentiality*: e.g. take care with whom you share information from medical records. Make sure that you have clear guidelines for confidentiality, and develop policies for giving results of investigations.
- *Health gain*: e.g. target those who are most vulnerable to the adverse effects of sexual risk taking.
- *Coherent team*: e.g. communicate new systems and procedures effectively between all those individuals who make up your team.
- *Audit and evaluation*: e.g. undertake regular audits and act on the findings to improve the quality of care.

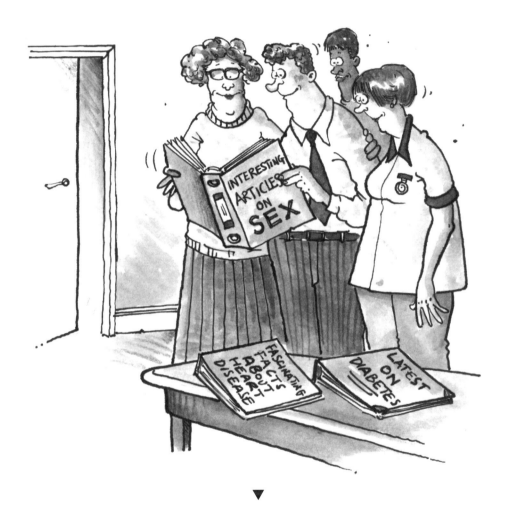

- *Meaningful involvement of patients and the public*: e.g. listen to and act on patients' comments about your clinical care or your services. Use patient groups.
- *Health promotion*: e.g. promote smoking cessation and prevention of sexual health risks, and obtain or write leaflets about sexual health matters.
- *Accountability and performance*: e.g. keep good records to demonstrate your own good practice.
- *Core requirements*: e.g. agree roles and responsibilities in the team for the various practice or workplace policies and tasks.
- *Risk management*: e.g. establish systems and procedures to identify, analyse and minimise the risks associated with, for example, repeat prescribing, over-investigation and unsafe working practices.

Now that you have completed the interactive reflection exercise in this chapter, transfer the information from this needs assessment to the empty templates. Use the personal development plan on pages 148–158 if you are working on your own learning plan, or the practice or workplace personal and professional development plan on pages 174–181 if you are working on a practice or workplace team learning plan. The conclusions reached at the end of each exercise will feature in the action plan. Don't forget to keep the evidence of your learning in your personal portfolio.

References

1 Greenhouse P (1994) A sexual health service under one roof: setting up sexual health services for women. *J Mat Child Health.* **19**: 228–83.

2 Chambers R and Wakley G (2000) *Making Clinical Governance Work for You.* Radcliffe Medical Press, Oxford.

3 Lilley R (1999) *Making Sense of Clinical Governance.* Radcliffe Medical Press, Oxford.

4 Wakley G, Chambers R and Field S (2000) *Continuing Professional Development: making it happen.* Radcliffe Medical Press, Oxford.

5 Stokes T (1997) Screening for *Chlamydia* in general practice: a literature review and summary of the evidence. *J Pub Health Med.* **19**: 222–32.

6 Stoke T, Schober P, Baker J *et al.* (members of the Leicestershire Chlamydia Guidelines Group) (1999) Evidence-based guidelines for the management of genital chlamydial infection in general practice. *Fam Pract.* **16**: 269–77.

7 Royal College of General Practitioners (2000) *Access to General Practice Based Primary Care.* Royal College of General Practitioners, London.

8 Dunning M, Abi-Aad G, Gilbert D *et al.* (1999) *Experience, Evidence and Everyday Practice.* King's Fund, London.

9 Chambers R (2000) *Involving Patients and the Public: how to do it better.* Radcliffe Medical Press, Oxford.

10 Department of Health (1997) *Report of the Review of Patient-identifiable Information.* In: The Caldicott Committee Report. Department of Health, London.

11 Donald P (2000) Promoting the local ownership of guidelines. *Guidelines Pract.* **3**: 17.

12 Muir Gray JA (1997) *Evidence-Based Healthcare.* Churchill Livingstone, Edinburgh.

13 Barton S (ed.) (2001) *Clinical Evidence. Issue 5.* BMJ Publishing Group, London.

14 Holland J, Ramazanoglu C and Scott S (1990) *Women, Risk and AIDS Project Papers 1–8.* Tufnell Press, London.

15 Bandolier (1999) Condom failure. *Bandolier.* **June**: 64.

16 Hannaford P and Webb A (1996) Evidence-guided prescribing of oral contraceptives. *Contraception.* **54**: 125–9.

17 Mohanna K and Chambers R (2001) *Risk Matters in Healthcare: communicating, explaining and managing risk.* Radcliffe Medical Press, Oxford.

CHAPTER 2

Opening the dialogue on sexual matters: keeping it confidential

Getting to see the health professional

This can often be the first hurdle for patients. The layout of the reception area may cause difficulties if patients at the desk can be overheard by others standing behind them. Clerks or receptionists often ask patients why they need an appointment, so that they can help by directing them to the appropriate person or clinic, or can make them an appointment of appropriate length. This can be very off-putting if you are a patient with a condition about which you feel embarrassed – whether it is your piles, your weight or your penile discharge! Sometimes receptionists have been placed in the difficult position of having to ask intrusive questions because of decisions made by other members of the team.

Box 2.1

At a practice meeting the two part-time practice nurses had complained that they were over-booked and constantly running late. Procedures that took a long time, such as four-layer bandaging for leg ulcers or a diabetic check, were being booked into appointments more suitable for a quick blood-pressure check. After discussion they had drawn up a list showing how long each procedure took. The receptionists were to consult this when booking patients to see the nurses. After a couple of weeks, one of the GPs noticed that she was seeing many more patients for emergency contraception. When she enquired about this, she discovered that these patients did not wish to tell the receptionist why they needed to see the nurse, so they had booked in to see the doctor instead.

Management decisions or staffing problems can alter the way in which patients are booked into appointments, and can be a cause of embarrassment or loss of confidentiality.

Box 2.2

Because of a shortage of doctors, several experienced family planning nurses were asked to run some clinics at short notice. A manager told the clerks to ring the patients to find out why they were attending, so that those who were unsuitable for nurse-led management could be rebooked. The manager thought that she was being thoughtful by avoiding wasted journeys, and was shocked to receive a complaint from a patient that her confidentiality had been compromised. After investigation, telephone contact was discussed with patients as they registered at the clinic and a definite record of their wishes was made on the notes.

Small changes at the interface between public and reception staff can make life more comfortable for both. Using a physical layout of the desk such that only one person is in front of the receptionist, with the others waiting some distance behind him or her, is helpful. A roped-off queue (as used in many shops) can prevent conversations at the desk from being overheard by the rest of the queue. A separate room for taking personal details is ideal. Some clinics have experimented with asking the patients to complete their own personal details when they first register. This could easily be modified so that patients complete the details on a computer screen (with access security procedures in place). However, those with literacy or language problems may have problems and need sensitive help.

Reception staff are the 'shop window' of any clinic or practice. Without their help, health professionals and patients may never meet so that the services required can be provided. The staff need training and practice to feel confident about their ability to spot the nervous patient who is unsure who they wish to see. Use role play or case scenarios both to help to understand why the difficulties arise and to rehearse ways of overcoming them.

You could ask some patients to help in training staff with regard to maintaining confidentiality and dealing with accessibility dilemmas by using fictional or anonymous scenarios. Some practices and clinics have asked patients to test their systems – but staff might feel justifiably angry if this was done without preparation! Notices in the practice or clinic leaflet and in poster form (*see* Box 2.3) help to spell out the importance of confidentiality.

However, many people do not or cannot read notices, so that verbal reinforcement of the messages about confidentiality is essential. For example, staff need to tell patients who arrive with an accompanying person (as young people often do) that they can be seen on their own if they wish, and that consultations are confidential to them. Advice about how to obtain results of tests should always include information to the effect that results will only be given to the person concerned, and not to relatives or friends.

Box 2.3 A sample confidentiality statement (modified from *Confidentiality and Young People: a toolkit for general practice, primary care groups and trusts*[1])

Here to listen, not to tell
We provide a confidential service to all of our patients, including under-16s. This means that you can tell others about this visit, but we won't.

The only reason why we might have to consider passing on confidential information without your permission would be to protect you or someone else from very serious harm. We would always try to discuss this with you first.

If you are being treated elsewhere – for example, at a hospital or clinic – it is best if you allow the doctor or nurse there to inform the practice of any treatment you are receiving.

If you have any worries about confidentiality, please ask any member of staff.

Concerns about confidentiality are the commonest reason why young people do not attend general practices for help and advice about sexual matters and other health worries.[1] Make sure that everyone knows the requirements for giving advice and treatment to young people (*see* Box 2.4).

Box 2.4 Guidelines for giving advice and treatment to young people

The Fraser Guidelines (also known as the Gillick Guidelines) were drawn up after Lord Fraser stated in 1985 that a doctor can give contraceptive advice or treatment to a person under 16 years of age without parental consent, provided that the doctor is satisfied that:

- the young person will understand the advice
- the young person cannot be persuaded to tell their parents or allow the doctor to tell the parents that they are seeking contraceptive advice
- the young person is likely to begin or continue to have unprotected sex with or without contraceptive treatment
- the young person's physical or mental health is likely to suffer unless they receive contraceptive advice or treatment
- it is in the young person's best interest to give contraceptive advice or treatment.

Confidentiality training for staff can be undertaken within the practice or clinic, as a primary care organisation (PCO) or trust, or by using outside courses. It is sometimes impossible to get all of the staff together unless this can be done when the surgery or clinic is closed. All new staff should have an induction period that includes an introduction to the confidentiality policy in the practice or workplace. The employment of new staff is often a good time for existing staff to refresh their own skills (*see* Box 2.5).

Box 2.5 Confidentiality concerns

- Discuss with colleagues or at team meetings any problems that have occurred with regard to the confidentiality policy. It is worthwhile for the practice manager or designated receptionist to keep a log of these problems so that they can be discussed (suitably anonymised).
- Use critical incident analysis to discover why problems have arisen, especially if there has been an adverse event or complaint.
- Any new procedures that are introduced may involve confidentiality issues (e.g. giving test results or notifying patients of changes of appointments).

- The confidentiality policy should be reviewed regularly, and also after any significant event analysis.
- The publicity about the confidentiality policy should be clear to both staff and patients (e.g. statements about confidentiality in the practice or clinic leaflet, notices in the waiting-room, etc.).
- Feedback from patients and the public should be actively sought. Many patients do not realise the extent to which clinical information is shared between health professionals.
- Review the transfer of information to other health service providers, insurance companies, employers, etc., to justify whether patient-identifiable information is being provided within the confidentiality guidelines.

You might like to take a look at how accessible your service is to members of the public who wish to use contraceptive or sexual health services. Reducing embarrassment at the reception desk might improve your services (and earn more money in contraceptive fees).

Box 2.6

Some practices use cards that patients can pick up from a box and hand to the receptionist to request an urgent consultation for emergency contraception. Other practices use a notice – for example, 'If you wish to obtain emergency contraception or discuss something confidentially with the practice nurse, please ask the receptionist if you can see Tracey'. Every new receptionist has to be told that 'Tracey' does not exist, but to contact the duty practice nurse to fit in the patient urgently.

Consider making the provision as flexible as possible. Some clinics see anyone who walks in, while other busier clinics may have to ask if the patient can wait to be fitted in after patients with appointments have been seen. Think about the following when making arrangements, and ask your patients what they prefer.

- Patients who book into a *general surgery session* do not have to state the reason for attending, either to the receptionist, or tacitly to the other patients in the waiting-area, or to people at work or at home who might want to know where they are going. The disadvantage is that lack of time or expertise may prevent adequate discussion if contraceptive or sexual health needs are complex.

- Patients who book into a *designated clinic* may be better able to state to the world that they are sexually active. They expect to receive more specialised attention and expertise at a clinic, and it is usually possible to give more time for more complex consultations. Giving the clinic a name other than 'Family Planning', and carrying out some other functions (such as cervical smears or well-person checks) may make it easier for patients to state that they wish to attend that clinic. Many clinics for young people have names thought up by the young people themselves, and they often offer other services in addition to contraception and sexual health services.
- Arrangements for *emergency contraception* need to be clear to patients and reception staff as well as the health professionals concerned. Notices about the time limits need to be prominently displayed (*see* Box 2.7). The reception staff need training to help them to recognise the need for rapid action. They require written instructions and available appointments with the doctor or nurse. Nurses are often in the surgery or clinic for longer than a doctor who may be out on visits or unavailable due to other commitments. A patient group directive, so that nurses feel confident to act independently, can extend the availability of emergency contraception by allowing them to give advice and prescribe emergency contraception. Surgeries or clinics can hold stocks of emergency contraceptive pills to issue to patients under a group directive.

Box 2.7 Example of a notice about emergency contraception

Emergency contraception is still available here free of charge.

- The hormonal (pill) method can be used up to 72 hours after unprotected intercourse.
- The intrauterine device (IUD or coil) can be used up to 5 days after unprotected intercourse – or sometimes later depending on your menstrual cycle.

Please ask for advice as soon as you realise that you are at risk.

If the clinic is closed, ring the sexual health helpline

on . . . . for your nearest open clinic.

- *Fears about a potential lack of confidentiality* prevent many people from consulting their own doctor or practice nurse about sexual health matters. Even at clinics away from their home area, people fear that their details will be passed on without their consent.

Practices and clinics need to consider both how to record information and how to control who has access to that information. Teenagers often believe that their details will be divulged to parents or other adults who they fear will be critical of them. Clear messages about confidentiality help to allay these anxieties.

- *Choice of access* to different types of provision can also improve access to sexual health advice. General practices that wish to provide specialist or more general contraceptive services can display notices that welcome all patients for registration for contraceptive services alone, and make it clear that they do not need to register for general medical services at that surgery. They can display the access arrangements for other clinics – a service that is especially welcome to patients if the alternatives are open at times when the surgery premises are closed. Community sexual health services in many areas provide a variety of access points, ranging from clinics run from shop premises that are open until late, to youth clubs, mobile buses, and outreach condom distribution on the streets in areas used by prostitutes.

Box 2.8

In North Staffordshire nurses trained in family planning are extending their roles by operating a 'clinic-in-a-box'. They go to settings where other facilities for young people are available (e.g. coffee bar, snooker, table tennis, etc.), and they take supplies of condoms, emergency and oral contraception, leaflets and other information. They are available to listen and give advice, and they can prescribe under group directives. The young people feel that they are 'on their own ground' and are often much more forthcoming than in more traditional 'medical' settings. This provision is particularly useful for engaging the attention of young men.

Why we need to take a sexual history

Most health professionals have had little training in taking a sexual history, diagnosing sexually transmitted infections or helping patients with simple sexual problems. Unease about discussing the area of sexuality can discourage practitioners from even approaching the subject.

In *A Survey of the UK Population* published by the Health Education Authority,[2] about one-third of informants who expressed an opinion

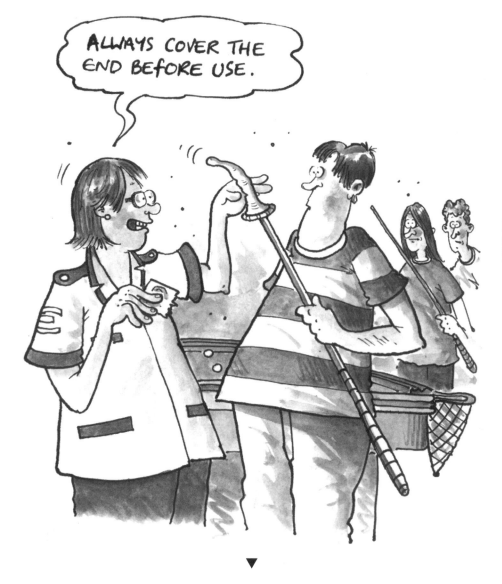

found sexual problems either difficult or impossible to discuss with their doctor. In order for them to feel able to broach the subject, patients need to feel that doctors and nurses are approachable and that they will not be judgemental.

The general public think that:

- health professionals are the appropriate people to approach with problems concerning their sexuality or sexually transmitted diseases
- health professionals will have the knowledge and skills to help them.

They hope that health staff will be professional and non-judgemental in their attitudes. Patients often present their problems in disguise out of fear that they will be criticised or condemned. We all recognise the scenario of a patient leaving after a consultation with a puzzled nurse or doctor, who is wondering why the patient had attended.

The health professional is usually the first person to be consulted when patients have problems with their sexuality or a sexually transmitted disease. It is important that they do not fail to discover the reason for the consultation, as that situation not only leaves the problem unresolved, but may also be harmful to patients and their sexual partners.

An anonymous postal general health survey in four general practices found that 44% of men and 36% of women reported that they had sexual dysfunctions (of various types), and 23% of men and 15% of women would like help for their problems.[3] The general practitioner was the person most of them wanted to approach, with women being more likely to want help from someone of the same sex.

Sex has become a common topic of discussion in the media, and is now mentioned much more frequently in social conversation. There is more openness about sexual problems and sexually transmitted diseases. Fear of AIDs, knowledge of herpes, and expectations of a rewarding sex life all cause patients to seek advice and help. Patients are more willing to bring their sexual health problems to health professionals than they were in the past, and they expect to benefit from professional expertise.

Increasingly, pro-active preventive medical health promotion is expected, rather than reactive illness care. Sexuality and its problems are more likely to be encountered when screening for cervical cancer, giving contraceptive advice, or discussing mammography or testicular self-examination. The prevention of transmission of common infections such as chlamydia, the prevention of pelvic inflammatory disease in young women, and the detection of subclinical sexually transmitted diseases in men are challenges which health professionals have barely started to tackle.

Why we have problems taking a sexual history

Doctors and nurses often say that they have avoided asking questions in order to avoid embarrassing patients. However, whose embarrassment are they really preventing?

In order to offer a good standard of professional care, we often need to ask intimate questions. For example, we have no difficulty in asking 'When did you last open your bowels?' or 'Are your motions runny?'. We ask 'When was your last period?', and 'Do you lose blood clots?' or 'Do you have to get up at night to pass water?' – not subjects that are usually discussed in a social context.

Asking patients to tell us about their sexuality seems somehow different, as if we are being voyeuristic and intrusive. It is often our own reluctance and our own unfamiliarity with the subject that makes it seem uncomfortable. Practise asking 'Do you have a sexual partner?' or 'Are there any problems when you have sex?', so that as part of normal history taking such questions become familiar and non-threatening.

One paper identified three main reasons for the difficulties encountered when taking sexual histories:[4]

- a belief that a sexual history was not relevant to the complaint
- embarrassment
- feeling inadequately trained to deal with the information obtained.

The first reason begs the question of how you know that a sexual history is not relevant if you have not asked anything about it. Training and practice will improve the other two.

Health professionals should be competent enough to obtain a satisfactory sexual history, even if they have no particular interest in that field and wish to refer the patient on to others. If they are to refer them on, it is not possible to know to whom the referral should be made without a good history.

For example, you should be able to take a good enough history to avoid referring inappropriately to:

- a urologist – *someone who says he has impotence, when in fact he is experiencing loss of interest in sex*
- the organisation Relate for relationship therapy – *a couple who say that they have gone off sex, when the problem is in fact postmenopausal atrophic vaginitis.*

An adequate referral letter can also aid the assessment of the urgency of the problem and the type of help that is needed, especially in cases where a waiting-list may be long.

If a sexually transmitted disease is a possible diagnosis, no examination can be accurate without a sexual history. The time of exposure to risk, the sites that may be affected, and any risk to others all need to be assessed.

If the doctor or nurse detects embarrassment in the patient when they are being asked intimate questions, they should become used to defusing the situation with humour or sympathy about the patient's discomfort. Avoidance of information gathering because it is emotionally charged leads to inadequate or inaccurate histories being obtained, and diagnosis and treatment of the problem will be impossible or incorrect. Inadequate histories with regard to sexual health risks, alcohol or other drug use, or problems with sexuality increase morbidity and mortality. Patients will also receive the message that they cannot talk openly with this health professional, and they often will not try to raise their concerns again.

Pitfalls when taking a sexual history

Taking a sexual history requires the same skills as other history taking, but there are additional difficulties. Both the patient and the health professional may be embarrassed because of unfamiliarity with open discussion of these matters. If the history is *not* taken in a competent way, inaccurate or misleading information may be recorded. The language used for sexual anatomy and sexual practices may not be common to both parties. Therefore particular care must be taken to establish whether you and the patient are talking about the same things. 'Making love' can mean anything from caressing or kissing to penile penetration of the vagina – which of these does the patient mean? 'Sleeping with' someone may mean sexual intercourse to you but just sleeping in the same bed to the patient. 'Vagina' means something quite specific to the health professional, but it may mean the vulva, the opening of the urethra, or the uterus, to the patient.

Assuming that the sexual partner is of the opposite sex is another pitfall. If it is not obvious from the name or the context, find out which it is by asking directly. Pat or Lesley could be either! 'Is Pat male or female?' signals to the patient that you are not likely to be shocked by what they say.

When to take a sexual history

It may also be necessary to explain to the patient why you need to know about their sexual history. It may not be obvious to them why you are inviting information on sexuality, if it is not in response to an overt presentation of a sexual problem. For example, you could say 'Some people find that going on to treatment for blood pressure affects their sexual life. Have you noticed any difference since you started on this treatment?'. You might enquire whether sexual intercourse is satisfactory after a hysterectomy or a prostatectomy, or after a myocardial infarct.

In a busy practice it is not possible to take a 'full history' from everyone. We all learn at an early stage in our training to focus on the presenting complaint and ask for information relevant to that. The history taking which we learned as students, going laboriously through each system, is simply impracticable and useless. If you listen without interrupting, most patients will tell you about the problem within between one and three minutes. Then, as with any other problem, checking that you have understood the problem and making supplementary enquiries completes the history of the complaint.

Consider the age of the patient

If you suspect sexual activity in children (e.g. for example because of vaginal discharge or perianal warts) this may have child protection or legal implications. You may need to think of referral at an early stage. Explaining that you do not have the necessary skills to sort out the problem which needs investigation is just as routine in this case as it would be for any other field in which you do not have expertise.

The older the child, the more appropriate it is to take a sexual history. To omit to take a sexual history from a teenager with cystitis, vulval or penile soreness or a genital rash might be negligent.

Most adults are not offended if you ask whether they are sexually active as part of a general enquiry. As we become older our perception of who is sexually active changes. Teenagers cannot believe that anyone over 40 years of age could still be sexually active, but the older we are, the more certain we become that sexuality continues into extreme old age. Most pensioners are pleased to be asked about this, although their activities may be restricted due to lack of available partners or infirmity.

Gender and setting

Women attend primary care more often than men. It is often easier to obtain a sexual history because they attend for contraception, care during pregnancies, and intimate examinations such as cervical smears. Men between 16 and 50 years of age attend primary care infrequently and often for urgent conditions such as accidents and intercurrent infections. You would not discuss sexual health promotion at such consultations (unless there was a clear link to their sexual lives, such as a sexually transmitted disease), but they could be asked to attend for a 'well-person' check.

Opportunities such as 'well-person' checks, the registration medical for new patients, or a consultation for travel immunisations may provide the perfect opportunity for dealing with sexual health promotion and enquiries about contraception or sexual health problems.

'Well-person' consultations

It is relatively simple to add sexual health-screening questions to a general medical history taken in the context of a 'well-person' check. In women, information often flows naturally from questions about contraception, pregnancies or gynaecological conditions. In men, urological complaints or bowel disorders may provide a useful starting point. You may want to introduce the subject by asking whether the patient lives alone or with a partner, and then move on to the particular as you did with other systematic enquiries. You might ask whether they have any problems with their sex life, if the contraceptive method used (if any) is satisfactory, and if there has been any change in partner recently.

Physical disability

The media projects an image of sexual activity being for the young and attractive. However, people with physical disabilities have the same rights to fulfilling and safe sexuality as everyone else. For young people with disabilities, sex education, information, family planning and advice are less accessible. Audiotape or Braille information leaflets are even less common than those available in minority languages. Access to surgery premises or clinics is frequently difficult, and carers are protective and often treat the disabled as children with no sexual needs or desires. It is sometimes difficult for health professionals to consult privately with someone with a disability, because the carer brings them into the room and stays to assist, thus preventing private conversation. Consider how you could consult privately with a patient in a wheelchair in your consulting room or clinic, at the patient's home or in a residential or nursing home.

Mental handicap

Some of the difficulties listed above may also apply to people with mental handicap. It is often difficult to talk with a person with learning difficulties on their own, and their carer may often answer for them. The carer may be more embarrassed than either the patient or the health professional, and may prefer to deny that sexuality is the problem. Development of interest in sexual needs for the first time at an older age can lull the carer into a false sense of security – the development of adolescent interest in sexual activity at the age of 26 years can be quite a shock. Health professionals may find themselves dealing with the confusion of the carer as well as the patient's problem. Problems associated with lack of knowledge, slowness of comprehension and idiosyncratic names for parts of the body are all hurdles in the path of clear discussion of sexual health. Use pictures, models or even dolls to demonstrate what you are discussing, break each communication into shorter parts, and check after each section to ensure that both you and the patient understand what has been said.

Psychosocial problems

Anxiety, depression and relationship problems are often associated with sexual difficulties. Health professionals are aware that sexual desire will be lowered in depression. Most also know that anxiety may cause loss or inhibition of erection in men and loss of vaginal lubrication in women. Similarly, sexual incompatibility or inadequacy may cause or be associated with insomnia, emotional distress or partnership disputes. Asking how the partner feels about the emotional problem, or enquiring directly whether the condition has affected their sexual feelings and activity, is frequently helpful in establishing the extent – and sometimes the causes – of the current problem.

Contraceptive consultations

Most people do not want to use contraception. Their priority is to be able to have sexual relationships. In order for a couple to use contraceptives, the perceived disadvantages of using a method of contraception have to be outweighed by the need to avoid pregnancy. The wish to avoid a sexually transmitted disease is even less of a priority. Most decisions about sexual relationships are made privately, but in order to obtain most methods of contraception a health professional has to be involved. The more difficult it is to consult that health professional, the less likely the patient is to do so. Organising the delivery of contraceptive care is an important part of enabling people to choose, use and continue to use contraception.

Interviews for contraceptive advice need to concentrate on the needs of the patients. You should be helping patients to understand how their sexual behaviour and the choice of contraception affects the risk of sexually transmitted infections as well as pregnancy. Looking at the implications of sexual behaviour is very important both when choosing and using a suitable method to prevent both risks.

Box 2.9

It is dangerous to make assumptions. The woman who tells you that she is a housewife and mother may have a husband who travels to the Far East on business trips and takes sexual risks while he is away from home. Screening her for STIs before fitting her with an intrauterine device may be a wise precaution that you would not otherwise have thought about without taking a sexual history.

Reflection exercises

Exercise 2

Review how accessible your service is to patients. Patients may not be aware, or not sufficiently aware, of what you do provide. A check-list like the one shown in Box 2.10 may help you to think about how accessible and full your service is. You might discuss this with other colleagues – perhaps from a different practice or area – in order to gain a fresh perspective on the situation, or ask a couple of patients to help you to complete the check-list.

Box 2.10 Check-list for access and range of services for contraception and sexual health

	Yes	No	Unknown
Is there information about contraception and sexual health in the practice or clinic leaflet?			
Are the contraceptive services that the nurses offer clear and visible to patients?			
Do you have posters on the walls giving details of the services available from you and elsewhere?			
Is there a visible statement about confidentiality?			
Do sessions coincide with bus times or school finishing times?			
Do you have walk-in sessions?			
Are some sessions outside usual office hours (e.g. evenings or lunchtimes)?			
Do you have posters and leaflets about sexual health and different methods of contraception in the waiting area?			
Are all methods of contraception available and is this visibly stated to patients?			
If some methods are only available elsewhere from other services, is this visibly stated?			
Is it obvious that emergency contraception is available and how it can be obtained?			
Is there a relaxed atmosphere with a comfortable waiting area?			
Is there provision for patients to bring children (e.g. a safe area for play)?			
Are the receptionists able to put anxious patients at their ease and respect their privacy?			
Is it clearly stated that everyone is welcome regardless of sexual identity or practice, ethnic origin, disabilities or disadvantage?			
Can patients choose whether to see a male or female health professional?			
Can patients choose to see a particular health professional?			
Do people in your area know about your services (e.g. in local pharmacies, youth clubs, other clinics)?			

Box 2.11 Audit on confidentiality

	Yes	No	Unknown
The practice/clinic has a policy on confidentiality			
The practice/clinic has a written policy on confidentiality			
The policy includes advice on young people under 16 years of age			
The policy was reviewed at a practice meeting within the last 18 months			
New members of staff have to read and sign that they agree to adhere to the confidentiality policy			
There is a statement about confidentiality in the practice leaflet			
There is a statement about the special requirements for young people under 16 years of age in the practice/clinic information			
There are notices about confidentiality in the reception area			
There are notices about confidentiality in the waiting area			
There are notices about confidentiality in the consulting rooms			
Issues about confidentiality have been discussed as they arise at practice/service meetings in the last year			
Significant event auditing has included confidentiality issues in the last year			
Training is provided for receptionists and secretaries in how to apply the confidentiality policy			
Training is provided for nurses in how to apply the confidentiality policy			
Training is provided for doctors in how to apply the confidentiality policy			
Training is provided for other staff (e.g. district nurses, health visitors, cleaners) in how to apply the confidentiality policy			
Training is provided for temporary staff in how to apply the confidentiality policy			
The manager is responsible for the shortened confidentiality policy that is signed by staff such as cleaners and maintenance staff when they work at the practice/clinic			

Exercise 3

Audit confidentiality in your practice. A sample check-list that you could ask each member of staff to complete is shown in Box 2.11. If there are any deficiencies, draw up an action plan at a practice meeting, and re-audit after the changes have been made

Exercise 4

Arrange a study afternoon for all staff, or for selected members of staff, to discuss scenarios involving difficult confidentiality issues, especially those concerning young people. Useful scenarios are included in the *Confidentiality and Young People Toolkit*,[1] or you could collect your own (suitably anonymised).

Exercise 5

Find out if there is any local or national information on where teenagers think emergency contraception can be obtained and how they would like to access contraceptive advice and treatment when they need it. Use the information to look critically at your publicity and provision for this age group.

Now that you have completed one or more of the interactive reflection exercises in this chapter, transfer the information from this needs assessment to the empty templates Use the personal development plan on pages 148–158 if you are working on your own learning plan, or the practice or workplace personal and professional development plan on pages 174–181 if you are working on a practice or workplace team learning plan. The conclusions reached at the end of each exercise will feature in the action plan. Don't forget to keep the evidence of your learning in your personal portfolio.

References

1 Donovan C, Hadley A, Jones M *et al.* (2000) *Confidentiality and Young People: a toolkit for general practice, primary care groups and trusts.* Royal College of General Practitioners and The Brook Advisory Centre, London.

2 Health Education Authority (1995) *A Survey of the UK Population. Part I.* Health Education Authority, London.

3 Dunn KM, Croft PR and Hackett GI (1998) Sexual problems: a study of the prevalence and need for healthcare in the general population. *Fam Pract.* **15**: 519–24.

4 Merrill JM, Laux LF and Thornby JI (1990) Why doctors have difficulty with sex histories. *South Med J.* **83**: 613–17.

CHAPTER 3

Contraceptive provision and hormonal contraceptive methods

Pro-active service provision

If you do not know what method of contraception a patient is using, *ask*! It is not well known that patients can register with any general practice for contraceptive services separately from general medical services. This should be made clear at all practices that are prepared to make provision for patients to be registered for contraceptive services only. You may want to discuss a policy with neighbouring practices so that they do not feel that you are 'poaching patients' – but they may be quite pleased to hand over some provision. For example, the provision of emergency contraception outside GP consulting hours can be delegated with a patient group directive to suitably trained practice nurses, or a teenage drop-in clinic can be run with appropriately trained school nurses and back-up from the GPs if required. Some provision could be provided by a community clinic to cover the hours when the surgery is not open, or to provide methods used by a minority of patients for whom it would not be cost-effective to establish such provision in one surgery only.

Think about how you can:

- make sure your services are welcoming
- make provision for individuals, especially young people, to be seen quickly and at a time when they can attend
- ensure that confidentiality is clearly advertised
- counter the myths about contraception, the risks of getting pregnant and the idea that babies give you love back!
- help people to be assertive with each other and only to have sex when they want to do so

- find out what people need, when and how
- use language that people understand.

Box 3.1 Watch your language

Miss K, a rather prim-looking 22-year-old, came to a clinic to ask for a supply of condoms. The nurse took her history and found that she had just started on the pill from her GP. When she was offered 36 condoms she looked horrified and said she only wanted to use them instead of withdrawal for part of the week she was not taking the pill. She leaned towards the nurse and told her confidentially that she thought the GP should not have told her to use withdrawal during that week – she didn't think it was a reliable enough method for a doctor to recommend. It took some time for the nurse to explain how the pill worked – in plain language – and to untangle the notion that a 'withdrawal bleed' between packets was not the same as 'withdrawal' as a method of contraception.

Expertise in contraception

It makes sense for someone in the practice to have special expertise in this field which is subject to rapid changes and frequent media scares or to have ready access to someone with that expertise. The benefits of accurate information and best management cannot be underestimated in preventing unwanted pregnancies. Practices, primary care organisations, and hospital and community trusts need to consider how to employ the specialist skills of trained nurses and doctors to best advantage for the population and to maintain a high level of skill. A possible arrangement for providing services is shown in Table 3.1.

Initial training for the Diploma of the Faculty of Family Planning (DFFP) with a plan for regular updating should be within the remit of all general practitioners. Interested doctors will take the specialist training for the fitting of implants and intrauterine devices. Teams concerned with provision of services may want to discuss arrangements for those doctors with special training to provide services for all practices within a PCO. A practice may want to use the local family planning service to provide some or all of the specialist provision, including the management of problems and difficult clinical situations.

Table 3.1 Provision of contraceptive services

Level	Staff and premises	Examples of services
Primary care basic provision	Individual general practice teams including GPs, practice nurses, midwives, health visitors, school nurses. Young people's clinics. Complementary family planning or sexual health clinics in areas of need. Outreach provision (e.g. schools, youth clubs, care homes).	Mainly continuing and emergency hormonal contraception and condoms, with referral to, or provision of, intermediate care for other methods.
Intermediate care provision	A central venue for several general practices or for a PCO providing specialist GPs, nurses, expert family planning or sexual healthcare staff.	Long-acting contraception (e.g. IUDs, injections and implants), barriers, male sterilisation, management of some problems with contraceptive methods. Teaching provision for the Diploma of the Faculty of Family Planning (DFFP) and nursing certificates.
Secondary care provision	At a district hospital, or outreach at a clinic, for several PCOs providing family planning, sexual health, gynaecology and surgical specialists.	Problems with contraceptive methods, female sterilisation, difficult male sterilisation. Teaching provision for all.

You need to consider how the practical training for the DFFP will be organised. A combination of log-book training in general practice surgeries and in specialist clinics is probably ideal, but GP registrars should be encouraged to do most of their family planning and sexual health training while on the gynaecology part of their hospital rotation. Those involved in providing the training will need to take the Membership (MFFP) of the Faculty of Family Planning and Reproductive Health Care (of the Royal College of Obstetricians and Gynaecologists) as well as having training in adult education.

Nurses also need a qualification if they are to feel competent in managing the important role of counselling and teaching of contraceptive methods. The minimum training would be the theoretical course, ENB 9903 Foundation in Family Planning and Reproductive Sexual Health Care. At least one practice nurse in the practice team in a group practice should have the ENB 8103 – The Practice of Family Planning and Reproductive Health Care – to gain both theoretical and practical training in fertility control, sexuality, health promotion and health screening for contraceptive users. Experienced nurses with the ENB 8103 or its earlier equivalents will need to be available to teach other nurses (and doctors) and provide supervision of the practical aspects of the training. They can also act as resources and mentors for less experienced or knowledgeable nurses.

Much of the advice and routine management of contraceptive care in healthy patients can be undertaken by properly qualified and experienced practice nurses, school nurses, midwives and health visitors.

In some areas, contraceptive users are taking a role in teaching others about selected methods.[1] Consider the needs of other members of the practice team. The reception staff in particular need training and education so that they can answer the queries of patients from a good knowledge base, know the best ways to cater for their contraceptive needs, and how and where those contraceptive needs can be met.

Contraceptive consultations

Sexual activity is enjoyable for most people, but contraception is hardly a feast of delight. Unless the advantages of avoiding pregnancy are obvious and people wish to use a particular method, it will be abandoned. It is therefore important to address the following points.

- Discover the patient's ideas about contraception and also those of his or her partner.
- Use your check-list to select out any patients for whom that method would not be safe. A selected list is shown in Box 3.5 and a fuller summary list can be found in the *RCGP Handbook of Sexual Health in Primary Care*.[2]
- Negotiate an acceptable method.
- Teach the method using visual aids such as leaflets and models.
- Arrange how to obtain supplies, advise when to return routinely, and set up a safety-net in case things do not go to plan.
- You can use any spare time for health promotion (advice on safe sex, smoking, diet and exercise, etc.), but remember that the prime concern is the provision of contraception.

You may want to think about who does what, and how. It is tempting to regard contraceptive consultations as pleasant interludes from consultations with ill or difficult patients, that do not require much attention. If they are conducted poorly and patients leave with an inadequate grasp of how they should use the method, or with unanswered (or unasked) questions about it, an unwanted pregnancy may result.

Box 3.2

A 19-year-old attended a clinic because her period was 8 weeks late, and she had a positive pregnancy test. She had not taken the pill since seeing her doctor a few months earlier. She had been having headaches and was worried that she would have a stroke. She said that she had been unable to ask the doctor about it as 'he had almost written the prescription before I sat down'. Although her blood pressure had been checked, the assumption that she wished to continue with this method of contraception had been made – so the patient had just stopped taking the pills. The only other method she thought she could use was condoms. She and her partner could see no way they could continue with a pregnancy, and she was distraught at the prospect of a termination.

Special considerations for young people

The *Effective Health Care Bulletin* on preventing and reducing the adverse effects of unintended teenage pregnancies[3] gives several useful messages for those providing contraceptive and reproductive healthcare to teenagers.

1 'School-based sex education can be effective in reducing teenage pregnancy, especially when linked to contraceptive services.' Therefore consider how you can link with local schools and school nurses.
2 'Contraceptives are highly cost-effective and can result in significant savings when used properly.' Make sure that you have recent and accurate information yourself, and that you have the skills and resources to help young people to learn how to use contraception effectively.
3 'Increasing the availability of contraceptive clinic services for young people is associated with reduced pregnancy rates.' Make sure that you know about and publicise the availability of special teenage

clinics. Encourage the development of youth-orientated clinics in places that are accessible to teenagers and open at times when they can attend.

4 'Contraceptive services should be based on an assessment of local needs and ensure accessibility and confidentiality.' Teenagers who live in rural communities, or who are disadvantaged by disability, find it particularly difficult to access confidential contraceptive services.

Consultations with young people[4]

- Discuss the guidelines on confidentiality with all young people.
- Always give young people the option of being seen alone.
- Follow up more frequently initially in order to build trust and confidence.
- Pelvic examination should only be considered if pathology is expected.
- Know the local procedure for child protection in case you learn that a young person is at risk of suffering or significant harm.
- Know and follow the 'Fraser (Gillick) Rules' for advice and prescribing for those under 16 years of age (see Box 2.4).[5]

Cultural issues

Each individual or couple attending for advice on fertility control has a unique need. In addition to those considerations that arise from the medical history, others are derived from their particular ethnic, social, family and cultural backgrounds. The background of healthcare staff can give rise to conflicts with the belief systems of the patients whose contraceptive requirements they need to meet.

The first step is to understand our own beliefs and values and how they are based on our own culture and upbringing. Then we need to understand what the issues might be for others from different ethnic or cultural groups or communities. In particular, we need to guard against stereotyping.

Box 3.3

A nurse in training wished to write a case study of what she saw as a cultural issue for unmarried Muslim women. An unmarried woman had told the nurse that her mother believed she had a duty to look in her daughter's handbag and inspect her belongings. Because of this, she would not use the oral contraceptive pill, but she was willing to use the contraceptive injection as she could conceal her use of that method. It was pointed out to the nurse that many mothers believe that they should inspect their daughters' belongings, and that this was not unique to women of the Muslim faith. It would be more important to establish, for each patient, what the situation was for that individual.

This is not to say that learning about other people's religious and cultural beliefs is not useful. A framework of knowledge helps to build bridges and increase understanding. For example, the knowledge that some religions believe that life begins at fertilisation and not after implantation helps a health professional to explore a patient's beliefs before spending unproductive time discussing an unacceptable method of contraception. Similarly, knowing a little about religious festivals or observances helps you to understand a woman's reluctance to consider a contraceptive method that might cause bleeding at a time that would be unacceptable. You might want to make a start by reading a book,[6] or gather information from the patients whom you see. It may seem frustrating to someone from a 'liberated western culture' that a woman must return home to discuss what she is to do about contraception with her husband, or with her mother-in-law. Always be ready to admit your ignorance and ask for explanations. Understanding the religious or cultural aspects will help the health worker to accept the patient's behaviour or beliefs, and will help the individual to trust the health worker as respecting her particular needs. The patient is then more likely to trust other advice as being in her best interests, rather than as being a solution imposed on her from an alien set of values. Always find out what would be useful for a particular individual, and do not assume that the opinions of one person from a specific culture or religion tell you what another will need.

Box 3.4

An administrator of a family planning clinic was instructed by her employing community trust to put up direction notices in Punjabi after the trust had asked community leaders what was the commonest language spoken in that area. After finding out from the patients what languages they read and what they would prefer, she declined. She reported back to the trust that although quite a lot of the patients spoke Punjabi, not all of them could read it, and there were at least nine different languages spoken, as well as several dialects. The *patients* said that they would prefer the notices to be larger, not in capitals, in English, and illustrated with pictures where possible.

Many religions and political systems support procreation and disapprove of contraception, but personal needs and beliefs may be quite different. Most people decide for themselves how much notice they take of cultural or religious pronouncements, but they may experience guilt and difficulties because of ambivalent feelings.

Young women with little ambition or poor education may also either use no contraception at all or use it erratically because of feelings of powerlessness, or because they feel that the only thing that they can do well, or be valued for, is to have babies. In every consultation establish what the beliefs are for the woman or couple, so that the choice of method will be suitable for them at that time.

Choice of method

No one method will suit everyone, and people will choose different methods at different stages of their lives. No ideal method exists, and all methods fail – some more often than others. If it is important to avoid pregnancy, then a reliable method should be chosen. Keep a good up-to-date reference manual such as the Family Planning Association's *Contraceptive Handbook*[7] or *Contraception: your questions answered*[8] ready to consult when any problems or queries arise.

Choice of methods requiring medical intervention

Box 3.5 lists some of the more common situations that are encountered in primary care which might make you recommend one method above another. There are few contraindications to specific methods – most people who consult for contraception are healthy and can choose freely from the full range of methods. You might want to mention briefly all of the methods that are suitable for an individual, and then concentrate on the most favoured one(s) for a more detailed discussion of the benefits and disadvantages.

Box 3.5 Conditions that require caution when choosing contraception (adapted from information from the World Health Organization[9])

Condition	COC	POP	Injection	Implant	Intrauterine system (IUS)	Copper IUCD	Barrier
Smoker over 35 years of age	P*	✓	✓	✓	✓	✓	✓
Postpartum almost exclusive breastfeeding: Under 6 weeks 6 weeks to 6 months Over 6 months	CI* P ✓	✓ ✓ ✓	P ✓ ✓	P ✓ ✓	P ✓ ✓	P ✓ ✓	✓ ✓ ✓
Postpartum not almost exclusively breastfeeding	Start at 21 days after delivery	(P) (best started after 6 weeks to avoid confusion about cause of irregular bleeding)					✓
Past ectopic pregnancy	✓	P	✓	✓	P	✓	✓
Trophoblastic disease	Seek specialist advice, no hormones or IUCD while HCG levels are raised						✓
Diabetes without vascular problems	P	✓	✓	✓	✓	✓	✓
Diabetes with vascular problems	CI	(P)	P	(P)	(P)	✓	✓

Hypertension	CI	(P)	P	(P)	(P)	✓	✓
Valvular heart disease	Seek specialist advice: if on warfarin avoid COC Risk of bacterial endocarditis: avoid IUCD/IUS						✓
Stroke/deep vein thrombosis/ pulmonary embolism	CI	P	P	P	P	✓	✓
Headaches: Without focal symptoms	P	✓	✓	✓	✓	✓	✓
With focal symptoms	CI	(P)	(P)	(P)	(P)	✓	✓
Breast cancer	Seek specialist advice: usually no hormonal contraception until clear for 5 years					✓	✓
Undiagnosed vaginal bleeding	Make diagnosis first						✓
Uterus distorted by abnormalities	✓	✓	✓	✓	CI	CI	✓
Pelvic inflammatory disease	✓	✓	✓	✓	P	P	✓
Sexually transmitted disease: Current	✓	✓	✓	✓	CI	CI	✓
Extra risk	✓	✓	✓	✓	P	P	✓
Recurrent urinary infection	✓	✓	✓	✓	✓	✓	P
Liver disease or hormone-related cholestasis	CI	P	P	P	P	✓	✓
Sickle-cell disease (not trait)	P	✓	✓	✓	✓	P	✓
Immuno-suppressives	✓	✓	✓	✓	CI	CI	✓
Liver enzyme inducers	Extra risk of pregnancy: advice on increased dose required					✓	✓

P*, use is possible, but assess risk: benefit ratio carefully; (P), broadly usable, possible small extra risks; CI, contraindicated; ✓, safe to use.

The combined oral contraceptive (COC)

Failure rate: many figures have been quoted, ranging from 99.9% to 95%.[7] The Family Planning Association quotes 99% with consistent use.

The low failure rate, lack of interference with sexual activity and regular lighter periods associated with its use make this an attractive method. Improvement of acne with oestrogen-dominant pills is an important selling point to teenage girls! Record the history you take to exclude those who are unsuitable for hormonal contraception, and update it regularly. Specific conditions to consider are listed in Boxes 3.5 and 3.6.

Box 3.6 Conditions to consider when prescribing combined oral contraceptives[10]

Advantages and indications
- Excellent protection against pregnancy
- Prevention of iron deficiency by reduction of menstrual loss
- Reduction of dysmenorrhoea
- Reduced risk of ovarian and uterine cancer
- Protection against pelvic inflammatory disease
- Less benign breast disease
- Fewer functional ovarian cysts
- Reduction of ectopic pregnancy risk because ovulation is inhibited
- Probable reduction in endometriosis
- Fewer symptomatic fibroids
- Probable reduction in the risk of thyroid disease, rheumatoid arthritis and possibly also duodenal ulcers
- Reduction in acne with oestrogen-dominant pills

Disadvantages and contraindications
- Requires consistent regular action by an individual
- Increased risk of venous thromboembolic disease (*see* below)
- Increased risk of arterial disease in users who smoke or have other risk factors, and with increasing age
- Increases in blood pressure
- Possible increase in risk of breast cancer being diagnosed while on COCs and for up to ten years afterwards (but less risk of an advanced cancer being diagnosed)
- Possible risk of being a cofactor in the development of cervical cancer

- Possible increase in the (very rare) risk of liver tumours
- Possible increased risk of choriocarcinoma in the presence of active trophoblastic disease
- Often associated with a long list of 'minor' side-effects, including nausea, depression, weight gain, bloating, breast tenderness, and lassitude, which have not reached the level of significance in good-quality clinical trials

Venous thromboembolism risks (approximate values)[11]

In pregnancy	60 per 100 000
Healthy non-pregnant women	5 per 100 000
Second-generation COC	15 per 100 000
Third-generation COC	25 per 100 000

Types of COC[11]

Second generation	Containing levonorgestrel or norethisterone as the progestogen
Third generation	Containing desogestrel or gestodene as the progestogen
Low strength	Containing 20 micrograms of ethinylestradiol
Standard strength	Containing 30 or 35 micrograms of ethinylestradiol in a fixed dose throughout *or* 30/40 micrograms phased (variable) dose Biphasic or triphasic COCs are more complex to take but may provide better cycle control in some patients
High strength	Containing 50 micrograms of ethinylestradiol and used mainly for patients on liver-enzyme-inducing drugs

Most young women will have no contraindications to the use of COCs, and after taking a history and checking their blood pressure you can concentrate on making sure that they know how to use them. Do not assume that they will know – many people misunderstand, or remember incorrectly, information acquired when it was not so important.

Most people are generally uninterested in the long-term effects of COCs, but you should always ask whether they have any worries and discuss them seriously in order to prevent early discontinuation. It is often a better use of time to postpone any detailed discussion of cardiovascular risks, breast cancer and smoking until later visits, when this information can be assimilated and balanced against the benefits of COC. The best time to discuss concerns is whenever the patient presents them, but a brief discussion will ensure that they do not become too worried if they do read the packet insert!

Use the first consultation to convey essential information about how to take the pill and how to cope with the minor side-effects. If the woman can start the pill on the first day of her period, she will have taken enough hormone to prevent ovulation in the first pack. If she starts later it will be at least seven days before she is safe. After a first-trimester miscarriage or termination she should start without delay, but in the mid-trimester and after delivery (if not breastfeeding), delay until day 21 after delivery. This avoids the increased post-delivery thrombosis risk, but starts the hormones in sufficient time to prevent the first ovulation. If the patient is breastfeeding then a progestogen-only method would be preferable.

Build in a safety-net with regard to what the woman should do if she experiences any major change in general health or has any problems about which she is unsure. Ensure that she knows she should seek urgent advice if she experiences any of the following:

- sudden severe chest pain, breathlessness or cough with bloodstained sputum
- severe pain in the calf of a leg, which persists or is accompanied by swelling
- severe stomach pains
- unusual severe or prolonged headache, visual loss, marked numbness or weakness affecting part of the body, disturbance of hearing, speech or balance, or a seizure
- hepatitis or jaundice.

Missed pills

Information about missed pills requires frequent repetition and reinforcement with a leaflet. Emphasise the dangers of lengthening the pill-free week. By the end of the pill-free week, follicles may only be a couple of days away from being ripe enough to release the ovum, and only become quiescent on restarting the COC. Fortunately, this degree of activity only occurs in a few women, but nearly a quarter of women show some ovarian follicular activity by the seventh pill-free day. Seven

after this are required to return the ovary to full quiescence[12] – this
is the basis for the advice to use added contraception or abstinence for
seven days after a missed pill (see Figure 3.1 for a flow chart of advice for
missed pills).

Discuss interactions with other medication. Antibiotics may reduce
the absorption of oestrogen, so advise the woman to take extra
precautions while she is on antibiotics and for seven days afterwards.
If on long-term antibiotics, the gut flora return to normal after about
two weeks, so no extra precautions are needed after three weeks of use.
Some anticonvulsants (phenytoin, carbamazepine, topiramate and bar-
biturates) and St John's Wort increase liver enzymes and reduce the
effectiveness of hormonal medication. In this case, shorten the pill-free
interval to five days, or give three packs continuously without a break
(tricycling) or increase the dose of oestrogen to 50 to 90 micrograms.
Use alternative methods if more potent liver enzyme inducers such as
rifampicin or rifabutin are being given. Check with a specialist if other
less familiar drugs are being administered, especially for new HIV
treatments.

Some pills are produced in an every-day package with dummy pills
for the seven pill-free days. These have not been very popular in the UK,
mainly because of the risks associated with missed pills around that
hormone-free week and the complicated instructions that are needed if
pills are forgotten or vomited. Triphasic or biphasic pills need more
careful explanation with a demonstration pack. The woman may be put
at risk of breakthrough ovulation if she takes one pack immediately
after another, because of the drop in hormone level. Postponing a
withdrawal bleed for a holiday, or if a pill has been missed in the last
week, needs careful explanation with regard to which pills to select in
order to maintain the same level of hormones.

If the patient is a young woman who is living with her parents,
discuss where she will keep her pills. If she has to conceal them from
other family members she may be more likely to forget them. Building
in reminder mechanisms, such as keeping the packet with her clean
underwear or with her toothbrush, may aid regular pill taking.

Progestogen-only pill (POP)

This method has a failure rate of about 2–3% p.a. with consistent use.

The need to take the POP at a regular time makes the method less
attractive for the young or those with erratic lifestyles. However, do not
underestimate a woman's ability to take the pill consistently if she
chooses to use this method. POPs have to be taken at the same time

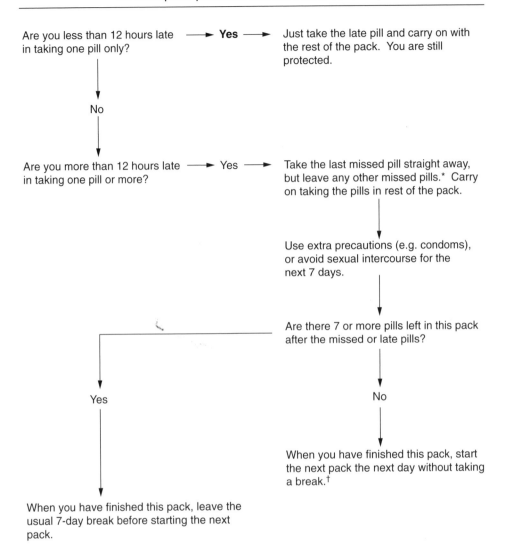

Are you less than 12 hours late in taking one pill only? → **Yes** → Just take the late pill and carry on with the rest of the pack. You are still protected.

No

Are you more than 12 hours late in taking one pill or more? → Yes → Take the last missed pill straight away, but leave any other missed pills.* Carry on taking the pills in rest of the pack.

Use extra precautions (e.g. condoms), or avoid sexual intercourse for the next 7 days.

Are there 7 or more pills left in this pack after the missed or late pills?

Yes

No

When you have finished this pack, start the next pack the next day without taking a break.†

When you have finished this pack, leave the usual 7-day break before starting the next pack.

* If you missed the pills in the first seven days of your pack, or you have missed four or more after you have taken the first seven pills, you may need emergency contraception *as well*. Talk to your nurse or doctor.

† If you are using a 28-day pack, you must identify the inactive pills and discard them in the above calculations. Ask your doctor or nurse for advice.

Figure 3.1: Advice on missed pills in a 21-day pack of pills.

every day without a break, and this sometimes makes them easier to remember than a pill with a week's break.

POPs are particularly suitable for those few women who have health risks. Although women with diabetes can take the COC, they usually have a regular lifestyle that is well suited to taking the POP. People with mobility problems (e.g. those in wheelchairs) can safely avoid the increased thrombosis risk associated with oestrogen by taking the POP.

However, be cautious about the use of the POP in obese women (i.e. those with a body mass index of more than 30 kg/m^2) who have an increased thrombosis risk with oestrogen. Weight over 70 kg appears to be associated with a higher failure rate for some progestogen-only methods[13] (although not demonstrated with the POP), so the use of two pills daily (although unlicensed) may need to be considered.

The POP is particularly suitable for women with good memories and regular lifestyles, and for those with contraindications to oestrogen (see Box 3.5 for cautions about use). Bear in mind that many of the exclusions for the POP have been drawn from extrapolation of evidence about COCs, and that you may need to seek expert advice in difficult clinical situations. The evidence for any need for caution in patients with thromboembolism, hypertension, diabetes mellitus or migraine is unsatisfactory.[11]

The POP works by keeping the cervical mucus in the post-ovulatory state, when sperm find it difficult to penetrate. The endometrium is thinner, and scantier irregular periods usually occur. In some women ovulation will be inhibited, and these women usually have amenorrhoea. Ovarian cysts can develop and cause pain, but they usually resolve spontaneously. The risk of breast cancer is thought to be of the same order as for COCs, and is very small.

Taking the POP

Advise women to take the POP every day at the same time. Help them to decide what is the best time for them. Blood levels will be highest about three hours after taking it, and then gradually fall, so the worst time to take the POP is just before expected intercourse, which for many people will be at night or in the early morning. Lunch-time or teatime is a good choice, but any time that can be regularly remembered is better than an imposed solution. Some women use alarm watches to remind them.

Box 3.7

An air stewardess decided that she would avoid the extra risk of thrombosis on long-haul flights by taking the POP. She decided to wear an alarm watch set to her pill-taking time, so that she would be reminded, regardless of which time zone she was in, to keep her pill taking a regular 24 hours apart.

Forgotten pills should be taken as soon as possible after they have been remembered, but extra precautions against pregnancy should be advised if the POP is forgotten for more than three hours. Standard advice (to harmonise with that for COCs) is that extra precautions (i.e. abstinence or condoms) should be used for seven days.

Interactions with hepatic-enzyme-inducing drugs are the same as for COCs, but antibiotics have no effect on absorption and blood levels.

Injectable progestogens

The failure rate of this method is less than 1% p.a. if repeated at the recommended intervals.

Depo-Provera (medroxyprogesterone acetate) and Noristerat (nor-ethisterone oenanthate) are extremely effective contraceptives. Injections are particularly suitable for women with heavy periods, for those who find it difficult to remember to take pills, or after a failure of other methods. Injections are a useful method for those with pill storage difficulties, such as women who are homeless, living in hostels or sharing a room with others. Women with learning difficulties or with disabilities who have problems in managing hygiene during their periods may welcome the amenorrhoea or light menstrual loss that usually occurs.

Box 3.8

L has spina bifida and spends long periods of time in a wheelchair. She finds the light occasional periods associated with use of the injectable contraceptive very convenient. She still lives at home but spends some nights away with her boyfriend, who also has a

---

physical disability. His mother does not mind them sleeping together, but L's mother still treats her like a child and does not approve, although L is now 22 years old. L prefers a method of contraception that her mother does not need to know about.

Give the injection within the first five days after the first day of the period and continue at 12-week (Depo-Provera) or 8-week (Noristerat) intervals.

Counselling about the usual infrequent or absent periods and the management of early irregular bleeding (see Box 3.9) is important for ensuring good continuation rates. You must also ensure that women have had ample opportunity to discuss any fears or queries about the method before giving an injection, as it cannot be discontinued by the user if she has second thoughts later! In the UK, Noristerat is only licensed for short-term use, but it is often used long term by those women who prefer it, perhaps because of the lesser risk of weight gain, or the slightly different side-effect profile of norethisterone. Most women prefer the less frequent injections of Depo-Provera.

Box 3.9 Management of bleeding problems with injectable contraceptives

1 Clarify the extent of bleeding.
2 Consider other causes (chlamydia, cervical ectopy, etc.).
3 Within 4–8 weeks of the last injection, consider using the combined pill (COC) for 21 days.*
4 Eight or more weeks after the last injection, consider a repeat injection.*
5 Consider alternative methods of contraception if this method is unacceptable.

* Evidence for these routines is lacking, but they are commonly followed.

Injectable contraceptives have no appreciable effect on the risk of thrombosis or a rise in blood pressure levels. It is suggested that they can be used in women with focal migraine[14] (who must avoid the combined oral contraceptive).

About 10% of women on Depo-Provera stay the same weight and 20–25% lose weight. It is common to gain some weight – the mean weight gain after 12 months is 2 kg, and after 5.5 years it is 9 kg,[14] representing slightly more than the average over this period of time in this age group. Noristerat users seem to show comparatively less weight gain, but good evidence for this is lacking.

The concern that bone density might be reduced in long-term users of Depo-Provera has been partially allayed by recent studies which showed no significant difference between users and the normal population mean. However, the combined oral contraceptive would be protective for those at extra risk of osteoporosis if there are no contraindications to the use of oestrogen.

The evidence concerning return to full fertility after discontinuation of Depo-Provera has recently been updated. It used to be thought that return to full fertility was considerably delayed. However, recent studies show no delay once the effect of the last injection has been eliminated (after 12 weeks). Comparative studies of the combined oral contraceptive pill, the intrauterine device and Depo-Provera give a delay to first ovulation of less than 30 days for all of these methods.[14] This has important implications for reinstated fertility if the woman is late attending for her next injection.

Consider reducing the interval between injections if a woman often attends late for her injection. The World Health Organization advises that both Depo-Provera and Noristerat injections can be given up to 2 weeks late, but the licence for Depo-Provera in the UK gives a margin of only 12 weeks and 5 days. After that you might offer emergency contraception if the woman has had unprotected intercourse. It is important to establish that pregnancy has not occurred before restarting the injection.

Emergency contraception

Make sure that *all* staff and patients know how to obtain emergency contraception and the time limits involved. You may need to put up notices informing patients that emergency contraception is still available from your practice on the NHS, as many patients have heard about the new arrangements for purchasing supplies from pharmacies. You can increase availability by using patient group directives so that suitably trained nurses can see patients and prescribe when a doctor is unavailable. Box 3.10 contains guidelines[15] that can be used as a basis for protocol production.

Box 3.10 Minimum information to be recorded in the notes prior to prescribing oral post-coital contraception

- Date of last menstrual period
- Usual cycle length
- Date and time of unprotected sexual intercourse (UPSI)
- Day of cycle of UPSI
- Any other UPSI since last menstrual period
- Options discussed (oral/IUD)
- Any interacting medication
- Current liver disease
- History of thromboembolism*
- Focal migraine at time when post-coital contraceptive is required*

Counselling should include the following:

- nausea or vomiting
- mode of action
- failure rate
- side-effects
- timing of next period
- action to take if next period does not occur on time
- discussion of future contraception needs.

Vomiting after taking emergency combined oral contraception
If the patient vomits within 2 hours of taking either dose of the pills, she should be advised to seek further medical advice. Domperidone 10 mg can be used to prevent vomiting.

Issuing guidelines
- Negotiate the time of the first and second dose and write them down.
- Go through the emergency contraceptive leaflet with the patient.
- Make follow-up arrangements or advise return one week after the expected date of the next period.
- Record what emergency contraception has been given or prescribed.

* Not a contraindication to progestogen-only method.

Table 3.2 Comparison of effectiveness of emergency contraception

Coitus to treatment interval	Percentage of expected pregnancies prevented by emergency contraception	
	Combined oestrogen/ progestogen	Progestogen-only
24 hours or less	77	95
25–48 hours	36	85
49–72 hours	31	58

The two hormonal methods, Levonelle-2 and Schering PC4, can be used up to 72 hours after unprotected intercourse, but the earlier the better. Levonelle-2 only contains progestogen and has a lower rate of nausea and vomiting than Schering PC4, which contains both oestrogen and progestogen. In trials comparing the two methods,[16] the progestogen-only method had a lower failure rate than the combined pill, especially within 24 hours of unprotected sex (see Table 3.2). Levonelle-2 is extremely safe and has minimal side-effects. There seems to be little justification for using Schering PC4 (despite the lower price).

Levonelle-2 is the name of the preparation prescribed by a doctor or nurse. Levonelle, with an identical formulation, is now available over the counter after a consultation with a pharmacist.

Multiple episodes of unprotected intercourse, even within the time limits, will increase the risk of pregnancy.

Don't forget that larger doses of hormone (probably three pills of PC4 twice or two pills of Levonelle-2 twice) are necessary for patients on hepatic enzyme inducers such as phenytoin or carbamazepine to obtain the same blood levels. Consider an intrauterine device if rifampicin is being taken, because it is such a potent, long-lasting enzyme inducer.

Another method of contraception, such as a barrier method (condom or cap) or abstinence, should usually be advised until the onset of the next period. Opinions vary as to how to restart the COC or POP pills after the use of emergency contraception, and there is no evidence to guide us. Most practitioners advise patients to continue with the pack and to take additional precautions for seven days as for the missed pill rules (see Figure 3.1), but some prefer to advise the use of other methods until the next period arrives and then restarting with a new pack. You may wish to take an individual decision based on the relative risks of each method and the number of pills that remain in the pack. However, there is no evidence that taking COC or POP pills when pregnant increases the risk of fetal malformations if the woman decides to continue with an initially undesired pregnancy.

Intrauterine device (IUD)

The insertion of a copper IUD up to 5 days after unprotected intercourse has an even lower failure rate (0.1%) than hormonal emergency contraception. It can be used up to 5 days after the calculated date of ovulation. This is calculated as day 19 of a 28-day cycle, counting day 1 as the first day of bleeding, and it successfully prevents implantation. The IUD can either be removed at the next menstruation if it is not required, or it can be retained for continuing contraception (*see* Chapter 4 for a more detailed discussion of IUDs).

Sexually transmitted infections (STIs)

Pregnancy is only one of the risk factors associated with unprotected intercourse. The latter also involves exposure to possible infection, so informed consent for screening is required, especially if an intrauterine contraceptive device is to be fitted. STIs will rarely be symptomatic by the time someone is seen for emergency contraception, if they become symptomatic at all (*see* Chapters 6 and 7).

Pharmacy availability of emergency contraception

Women who have attended a pharmacy to obtain Levonelle are still at risk of developing a STI and may not be counselled about this at the time. Other disadvantages of obtaining emergency contraception from a pharmacy are the cost and the lack of confidentiality. Considerable efforts have been made to ensure that pharmacists have adequate training before providing this service, but provision is patchy.

Box 3.11

An off-duty health visitor saw a young woman asking for Levonelle in a chemist's shop one Saturday afternoon. The shop did not have a pharmacist trained in the provision of post-coital contraception, and the counter assistant advised the woman to ring a nearby chemist using the phone in the shop.

She did this in the shop, in full view and earshot of the other customers. Having discovered that she could obtain Levonelle there, she then had to ask the assistant for directions to the other shop. The health visitor followed the young woman out of the shop to find her outside in tears with embarrassment and anger.

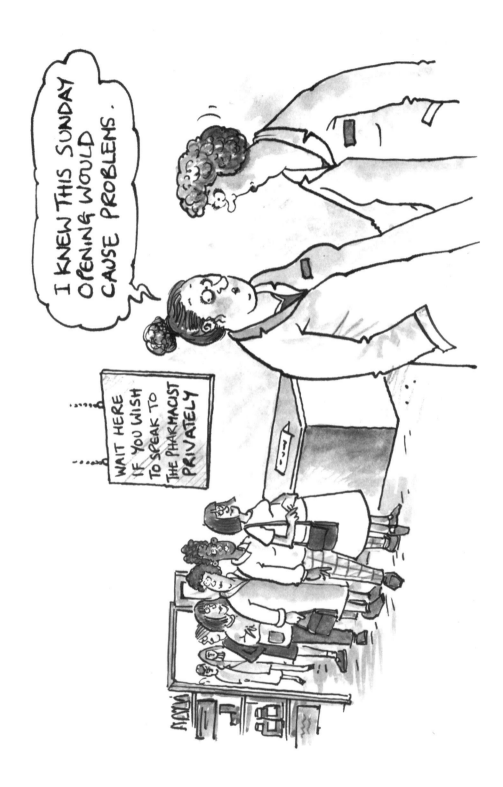

Women may also be tempted to use the method more frequently (cost permitting), as there is nothing to stop someone visiting different pharmacies several times in succession for supplies and lying about previous use of the method. However, this has also occasionally been experienced in family planning clinics, and is dependent on the patient's honesty.

The availability of counselling and provision of emergency contraception by pharmacies increases access to the method and can reduce the delay before access is obtained. The pharmacists and their staff increase their knowledge of local provision for contraceptive and sexual health advice, and can pass on this information to their customers. If you obtain a history to the effect that a woman has obtained a previous supply from a pharmacy, it is sensible to check that she is aware of her risk of STIs, and to offer screening as necessary.

Transferring to more reliable methods of contraception

Menstruation following hormonal emergency contraception may be delayed, especially if the drug was taken in the second half of the cycle. Standard advice is to check with a pregnancy test if the expected period is delayed by more than seven days. The COC or POP can be started once the menstrual flow is confirmed. Most practitioners suggest starting on the second day of menstruation rather than the first day, and continuing with a barrier method until seven pills have been taken. If the woman is starting on an injectable contraceptive or an implant (*see* Chapter 4), it is even more important to establish the absence of pregnancy, as there may be no alert raised by the subsequent absence of periods. If it is not convenient to delay the injection until the fourth or fifth day of a good flow of menstruation, or if the flow is light, you may wish to check by performing a pregnancy test before giving the injection.

An IUD that has been fitted as an emergency procedure can be continued as the regular method of contraception if this is desired and the method is suitable for the individual.

Reflection exercises

Exercise 6

Health professionals can use audit to check that they are providing good-quality contraceptive services for the majority of their patients.[17] If claims/attendances for contraceptive services in a practice or clinic are low, completion of claim forms/attendance records may be incorrect or the staff may need more training in sexual health and contraception. Are the receptionists sensitive to the needs of patients who are seeking contraceptive care? Try introducing a card system[18] (whereby women who need emergency contraception show a card to the receptionist) to avoid delay. Make sure that choice for patients is maintained, and that staff (receptionists as well as health professionals) in general practices and clinics know the various ways of obtaining contraceptive care from other sites. Lists of clinics and willingness to see patients who are not registered for 'contraceptive-only' consultations are important factors in improving access, and staff should have a good level of knowledge about where emergency contraception can be obtained at times when they themselves are not available.

Exercise 7

You could liaise with a local school to ask teenagers and teachers who have not previously used contraceptive services in your area to find out what is available and where, and how quickly they could obtain contraception if they required it urgently. Use this information to target your publicity about services more accurately.

Exercise 8

Audit the contraceptive records of those patients who are on the COC. You might want to set some standards, such as those in Box 3.12.

Discuss any shortfall at the practice team meeting and decide how any problems could be put right. Arrange to re-audit 12 months later (or earlier if there is a major problem, such as no blood pressure recordings).

Box 3.12 Standards for recording of COC consultation

Blood pressure recorded before first prescription	100%
Blood pressure recorded in the last 12 months for continuing use	100%
Smoking history recorded	100%
Contraindications recorded as excluded	90%
Other methods discussed at any consultation in the last 12 months	60%
Record that method has been taught	90%
Knowledge of missed pill rules checked, etc.	80%

Exercise 9

Examine a critical incident involving an unwanted pregnancy and discuss at a team meeting how the patient could have been managed better. Were there any indications that contraceptive needs were not being met (e.g. a consultation for urinary tract infection in a 14-year-old or a sudden increase in attendances for trivial matters)? You might want to take one incident involving a girl aged under 16 years and another in a woman aged over 35 years to determine whether the service needs are different.

Exercise 10

A practice or clinic team could collect information about uptake of contraceptive services in both clinics and general practices by teenagers from postcodes in their areas to compare with national levels. If the uptake is below average, strategies for improving access to services are needed.

Now that you have completed one or more of the interactive reflection exercises in this chapter, transfer the information from this needs assessment to the empty templates. Use the personal development plan on pages 148–158 if you are working on your own learning plan, or the practice or workplace personal and professional development plan on pages 174–181 if you are working on a practice or workplace team learning plan. The conclusions reached at the end of each exercise will feature in the action plan. Don't forget to keep the evidence of your learning in your personal portfolio.

References

1 Pickard S, Baraitser P and Herns M (2000) *Can laywomen provide quality, patient-centred training for doctors?* Poster presentation. In: Abstract of Proceedings of Annual Symposium, Faculty of Family Planning of the Royal College of Obstetricians and Gynaecologists.

2 Carter Y, Moss C and Weyman A (eds) (1998) *RCGP Handbook of Sexual Health in Primary Care.* Royal College of General Practitioners, London.

3 NHS Centre for Reviews and Dissemination (1997) Preventing and reducing the adverse effects of unintended teenage pregnancies. *Effect Health Care Bull.* **3**: 1–12.

4 Cooper P, Diamond I, High S and Pearson S (1994) A comparison of family planning provision: general practice and family planning clinics. *Br J Fam Plan.* **19**: 263–9.

5 Guidance issued jointly on confidentiality and people under 16 (1993) BMA, GMSC, Health Education Authority, Brook Advisory Centres, Family Planning Association and RCGP leaflet.

6 Schott J and Henley A (1996) *Culture, Religion and Childbearing in a Multiracial Society.* Butterworth-Heinemann, Oxford.

7 Belfield T (1999) *Contraceptive Handbook* (3e). Family Planning Association, London.

8 Guillebaud J (1999) *Contraception: your questions answered* (3e). Churchill Livingstone, London.

9 World Health Organisation (2000) *Improving Access to Quality Care in Family Planning.* World Health Organization, Geneva.

10 Hannaford P and Webb A (1996) Evidence-guided prescribing of oral contraceptives. *Contraception.* **54**: 125–9.

11 Joint Formulary Committee (2001) *British National Formulary.* BMA and Royal Pharmaceutical Society of Great Britain, London.

12 Korver T, Goorissen E and Guillebaud J (1995) The combined oral contraceptive pill: what advice should we give when pills are missed? *Br J Obstet Gynaecol.* **102**: 601–7.

13 Vessey M and Painter R (2001) Oral contraceptives and body weight: findings in a large cohort study. *Br J Fam Plan Reprod Health Care.* **27**: 90–1.

14 Bigrigg A, Evans M, Gbolade B *et al.* (1999) Depo-Provera. Position paper on clinical use, effectiveness and side-effects. *Br J Fam Plan.* **25**: 69–76.

15 Faculty of Family Planning and Reproductive Health Care (2000) Emergency contraception: recommendations for practice prepared on

behalf of the Faculty of Family Planning and Reproductive Health Care. *Br J Fam Plan.* **26**: 93–6.

16 Task Force on Post-Ovulatory Methods of Fertility Regulation (1998) Randomised controlled trial of levonorgestrel versus the Yuzpe regimen of combined oral contraceptives for emergency contraception. *Lancet.* **352**: 428–33.

17 Rowlands S (1997) *Managing Family Planning in General Practice.* Radcliffe Medical Press, Oxford.

18 Emergency Contraception Pack (1999) Posters, leaflets and credit cards for requesting emergency contraception are available from the Contraceptive Education Service at the Family Planning Association, 2–12 Pentonville Road, London N1 9FP; and www.fpsales.co.uk .

CHAPTER 4

Long-acting and non-hormonal methods of contraception

Introduction

Although your practice is unlikely to provide *all* methods of contraception, it is important to discuss some of the other methods. Too often it is assumed that people will want to use the combined oral contraceptive pill and condoms, or the injection, because these methods are the ones that health professionals would like them to use for maximum contraceptive efficacy. People frequently abandon a method that does not suit them or their lifestyle, and they risk pregnancy because they were unaware of other possibilities. If all possibilities have been considered, people are not left thinking 'There must be something better than this' or 'I'm not having sex often, so I won't bother with all this stuff'.

Abstinence

The effectiveness of this method is 100% if used reliably and 10–20% if not (i.e. the background risk of becoming pregnant if no contraceptive method is used).

Abstinence means choosing not to have sexual intercourse at all (not just sometimes!). This is very difficult when passions are running high in new relationships, and it requires a co-operative partner who agrees to it. Abstinence only works if both partners trust each other to abide by the rules. If one person cannot trust the other then complete avoidance of sexual touching is necessary. Abstinence can range from no body contact at all to holding hands, kissing and petting or even having oral sex. The important point is that there is no contact at all between the penis and the female genital area. The male produces ejaculate laden with sperm (and sometimes other undesirable things like infection) long before ejaculation. Advising someone about this method means discussing issues such as what other sexual release that couple might want (e.g. masturbation) and being able to discuss other forms of sexual expression that do not involve genital contact.

Abstinence is particularly suitable for people who are undecided about a sexual relationship, or who have (religious) beliefs about chastity, or if both partners agree about abstinence. It is not ideal, but possible, to use a combination of periodic abstinence and so-called 'natural methods'. Compared with the usual sex education programmes, abstinence programmes in schools were not shown to have any additional effect in delaying sexual activity or reducing pregnancy.[1] Abstinence cannot be imposed on people against their will!

Periodic abstinence or 'natural methods'

Failure rates are difficult to establish because of the varying application of these methods, but they are usually quoted as being between 2% and 20% yearly.

A number of indicators can be used to inform a couple of the stage of the cycle when they are most fertile. The more indicators that are used, the more reliable is the method. It depends on *predicting* ovulation (which *usually* occurs about 12–16 days *before* the next menstrual period in a regular cycle). Using cycle length alone (the calendar method) is the least reliable way of predicting ovulation, but it can be combined with the following:

- waking body temperature
- cervical secretions (mucus)
- fertility devices that measure hormone changes (e.g. 'Persona').

All of these methods need to be accurately taught over several cycles for best practice, and they depend on the couple abstaining from sexual intercourse during the fertile days. People often ask about this method and have poor information about its effectiveness or otherwise. After full counselling, they often decide that it is not a method that they can rely upon. Using a fertility predictor such as Persona is also rather expensive, as it is not available on the NHS. Restriction of sexual intercourse to the time after ovulation has occurred makes it a much more reliable method, but requires considerable self-control by both partners.

The other 'natural method' which is often neglected, is *fully* breastfeeding (no supplements, and on demand day and night) up to six months after delivery and before menstruation has restarted. This is only suitable for baby spacing for those who are in stable, well-supported relationships in which an unplanned pregnancy is not unwelcome, but is better than *nothing* for an unsupported single mother who is embarking on a new relationship!

Withdrawal (coitus interruptus)

It is difficult to establish the failure rate. Studies have mainly been conducted on couples in stable long-term relationships in whom the fertility rate does not seem to be increased compared with groups that use barrier methods.

Withdrawal is a commonly used method, and is certainly better than no contraception at all in an emergency. It should be more widely discussed, as many people who are just starting to engage in sexual activity have given no thought to contraception until after penetration. Withdrawal would certainly have an impact on teenage pregnancy rates if it was regarded as something at which young men should become expert!

The main disadvantage is the control necessary to withdraw before ejaculation. For many couples this appears to have no adverse psychological effects, but others complain that it leaves them feeling incomplete or frustrated. Predicting the moment of orgasm may be particularly difficult for young men, who often have premature ejaculation and have yet to learn control over the mechanisms for delaying ejaculation. Some sperm may be present in the pre-ejaculate fluid, and this may contribute to the perceived high failure rate of the method.

There are many other more reliable contraceptive methods but this one is (sometimes) possible in an emergency! It should preferably be backed up by rapid access (within 24 hours if possible) to emergency contraceptive methods, and serious consideration of more long-term methods.

Progestogen implants

The failure rate of this method is very low, and it is probably as reliable as sterilisation (but it is a relatively new method, so we await more widespread use for definite results).

Norplant has now been discontinued by the manufacturers. The surgical insertion of six rods and their visibility in the skin of the upper arm deterred some women, while others wore them like a badge proclaiming their protection. They require removal by a doctor trained in the removal technique after five years of use.

Implanon, which was recently introduced, has only one rod (about the size of a hairgrip), so insertion and removal are easier. It can be felt under the skin, but is less visible than Norplant as it lies in the groove between the muscles. It is inserted just beneath the skin on the upper arm under local anaesthetic with a special introducer. It should be inserted within five days of the first day of the period, or while other reliable contraception is being used. It can remain in place for three years and then be removed under local anaesthetic by making a small cut in the skin and pulling out the plastic carrier rod.

Good counselling about progestogenic side-effects, especially the irregular bleeding, reduces removal rates. Blood levels are similar to those obtained with the progestogen-only pills, and side-effects are about the same, but without the need for a good memory!

This method is particularly suitable for individuals who want a long-term, reliable method. It may be less acceptable if irregular periods are unwelcome or disliked, or for those who are afraid of minor surgical procedures. Contraindications are the same as for any progestogen-only method.

Intrauterine devices (IUDs)

The failure rate is less than 1% in the first year.[2]

Copper-bearing IUDs appear to act mainly by blocking fertilisation. Sperm transport is impaired and studies show that viable sperm are hardly ever found in the upper genital tract, in contrast to other methods in sexually active women.[3] The secondary protection from implantation blocking rarely has to come into action except when used for post-coital protection.

The risk of chlamydial infection and pelvic infection is increased in the young and in those who have had more than two partners in the last 12 months.[4] Consider taking swabs (with informed consent) before fitting an IUD, especially in higher-risk patients (see Chapters 5 and 6). The risks of infection with an IUD occur mainly in the first three weeks. Bacteria from the vagina may be taken into the uterus and cause endometritis or salpingitis during the fitting of the device. A sexual history and an estimate of the risks of changes of partner must be balanced against the effectiveness and ease of use of the method.

The choice of IUDs in general practice may be limited by which ones are on the drug tariff. Devices that have a surface area of copper of less than 300 mm^2 are associated with a higher pregnancy rate than those with a larger area of copper.

The Copper T380 series has low pregnancy rates, with the Multiload 375 running a close second. Recently, the CuT380S (Gyne T 380) has been discontinued. Replacements include the CuT380A (Tsafe 380A), which has an insertion fitting width of 6.6 mm, compared with 4.4 mm in the previous device, and no loading or depth device on the inserter tube. The Cu380Ag (Nova T 380Ag) is identical to the previous Nova T 200 except for extra copper on its stem, but it should give lower pregnancy rates. The confusing names for these devices mean that you should inspect the pack carefully before fitting, and record the type of device used carefully.

The Flexi-T 300 is introduced into the uterus with a simple push–pull action like the Multiload. Gynefix is a frameless device consisting of copper tubes that is fixed into the fundus of the uterus with a knot, and it requires special training to fit. New IUDs are being developed with similar technology.

All of these devices are usually removed and refitted after five years (except the Tsafe 380A, which has a licence for eight years). However, if the woman had the IUD fitted after the age of 40 years, it is normally removed after the menopause is definite (conventionally regarded as one year without periods after the age of 50 years, or two years without periods before the age of 50 years). Too frequent removal and refitting increases the risk of infection, expulsion and failure.

The Nova T 200 or the Multiload 250 are usually only regarded as suitable for short-term use because of their slightly higher pregnancy rate, but the Nova T 200 has a narrow inserter and is much easier to insert for post-coital use in women who have had no vaginal deliveries.

Pre-insertion counselling should cover the advantages of this method as well as how to recognise the signs of expulsion, perforation, infection and ectopic pregnancy. Modern devices cause only a small increase in the duration and heaviness of the regular menstrual loss, but irregular spotting is quite common in the first few months.

IUDs are more suitable for stable long-term relationships, for spacing pregnancies, and for long-term use after the family is complete.

The intrauterine system (IUS) Mirena

The failure rate is quoted as being 0.2 per 100 women years.[2]

The IUS is a T-shaped device with progesterone loaded on the upright stem. Its main effects are to reduce the endometrial thickness and maintain the cervical mucus in its post-ovulatory thickened state. Menstrual flow is markedly reduced making it an ideal contraceptive for women who usually have a heavy menstrual loss.

The introducer for fitting this device has recently been changed to make it simpler to use, but the IUS should only be fitted by health professionals who have been trained in its use.

Counselling before insertion should include advice about the expected menstrual pattern, namely frequent, sometimes continuous, light bleeding in the first three to six months, settling to very light occasional loss or amenorrhoea. Side-effects due to the progesterone, such as acne and bloating, may also occur during the first few months, but they usually settle down as the blood level falls to below one-third of the progesterone-only pill. Functional ovarian cysts may occur, but they usually resolve spontaneously.

The full efficacy of the IUS is manifested once the progesterone has exerted its effect. Because of the delay after fitting for full efficacy, it is not licensed for post-coital contraception, and you should insert it within the first seven days after the onset of the menstrual period.

Condoms

Failure rates are quoted as 3% for perfect use and 14% for typical use.[2]

Not all general practices are able to provide condoms free to the user, but health professionals should be aware of the types that are available. Different sizes and shapes suit different sizes and shapes of men. Health professionals should know where condoms can be obtained free to the user (e.g. at community clinics) and other sources of supply. It is useful to have some idea of the cost to the public as well. Recommend them additionally for protection against infection to those who are likely to change partners. Discuss with people how they can negotiate the use of condoms with a partner, and how to obtain emergency contraception in the event of a failure in their use.

Health professionals and providers of condoms need to be comfortable about discussing how a condom should be used and suggesting ways in which it can be incorporated into love play. The use of water-based lubricants (not lubricants containing oil, as this can weaken the latex) can reduce tearing and irritation as well as increasing sensitivity. It is even better to use a spermicide-containing lubricant that may further reduce the risk if spillage or tearing does occur. Don't believe that condoms burst – the average condom stretches to about 150 centimetres (five feet) long and can hold 16 pints of beer! Instruction should include holding the base of the condom after climax and before withdrawing to prevent spillage, and disposal of used condoms.

Female condoms (Femidom) need to be used carefully and the penis positioned so that it is covered by the closed-ended sac of the condom. They are rather expensive, but can be bought from a pharmacy with no need for medical intervention. They are disliked by some because of the 'plastic mac' feel, and they are noisy in use.

A proportion of both men and women dislike any form of barrier, be it a condom or a diaphragm (see below), as they feel that this distances them emotionally from their partner, or that it reduces sensitivity so that pleasure is diminished. However, some of the expressed dissatisfaction with barrier methods is due to myth rather than personal experience. Many of those who refuse to use barrier methods have never tried them and use the lack of sensitivity as an excuse to cover up other concerns. For example, they may have fears of losing the erection, of appearing foolish (because of lack of skill in putting it on), or of making the partner think that they are afraid of catching an infection.

Others welcome a method that reduces the messiness of ejaculation, or even prefer the emotional sense of distance that barriers produce, and may have difficulties if they then cease to use the barrier due to a need for a change of method or a desire for pregnancy.

Diaphragms and caps

Failure rates are 5% for perfect use and 21% for typical use.[2]

Having a diaphragm or cap fitted involves a vaginal examination, and this may deter some women. The diaphragm or cap must always be used together with a spermicide. Good teaching and practice are essential to ensure that the diaphragm and pool of spermicide cover the cervix. Health professionals who fit cervical caps should be competent to fit them accurately and be able to choose the right type for each individual.

The degree of organisation and forward planning required for reliable use makes diaphragms or caps a more suitable choice for those in stable long-term relationships. Patients also require access to (preferably private) washing facilities and convenient storage.

Sterilisation

Failure rates are as follows:

- *female*: between 1 and 5 per 1000 women, depending on the method used
- *male*: about 1 per 1000 men.

Late failure can occur. In women there is a risk of ectopic pregnancy in about one-third of the late failures. In men, failure can occur even after negative sperm counts. The incidence of late failure rates is quoted as ranging from 1 in 3000 to 1 in 7000.[5]

Ideally both partners should be involved in the decision, but the consent of the other partner is not required. There is a tendency for younger people (under 30 years of age) to regret the decision. Most male vasectomies are performed under local anaesthetic. Female sterilisation is usually performed under a short general anaesthetic using a laparoscope, but some operators offer the procedure under local anaesthesia. Laparoscopy may cause technical difficulties if the woman is obese or has had previous pelvic surgery or sepsis.

Other contraceptive precautions should be continued until the first period after a female sterilisation, or until two consecutive negative sperm counts have been obtained after a vasectomy.

Any causal relationship between vasectomy and testicular or prostate cancer has not been proven, and seems unlikely on biological and epidemiological grounds.[5]

Reflection exercises

Exercise 11

Use a significant event analysis of a patient attending for emergency contraception after the time limit for the hormonal method of post-coital contraception. Examine how she was managed in order to determine whether any changes to your provision for fitting of IUDs in an urgent situation are needed. Do more doctors need to be trained to fit IUDs? Would they fit IUDs often enough to maintain their skills if they were trained? Do you or your staff need more information about alternative venues where an emergency IUD can be fitted? Are any changes to your provision for hormonal contraception needed in order to avoid any delays produced by 'the system' rather than by individual patients?

Exercise 12

You could ask patients for feedback on how many methods of contraception they know about and whether they feel that they have enough information about the various alternatives after consulting you or your colleagues. This could be done by means of a questionnaire, focus groups or individual interviewing. Use the results to modify the way in which information about contraception is disseminated in your team, or to identify learning needs among the staff – or to congratulate the staff on how well they are doing!

Exercise 13

Use an attractively presented meeting with a popular speaker on some aspect of contraceptive provision to discover the knowledge gaps of the staff. A questionnaire with a prize for the first completely correct answer sheet will help you to tailor future training to the needs of the audience.

Now that you have completed one or more of the interactive reflection exercises in this chapter, transfer the information from this needs assessment to the empty templates. Use the personal development plan on pages 148–158 if you are working on your own learning plan, or the practice or workplace personal and professional development plan on pages 174–181 if you are working on a practice or workplace team learning plan. The conclusions reached at the end of each exercise will feature in the action plan. Don't forget to keep the evidence of your learning in your personal portfolio.

References

1 Cooper P, Diamond I, High S and Pearson S (1994) A comparison of family planning provision: general practice and family planning clinics. *Br J Fam Plan.* **19**: 263–9.

2 Trussel J (1988) Contraceptive efficacy. In: J Trussel, F Stewart, W Cates *et al.* (eds) *Contraceptive Technology* (17e). Ardent Media, New York.

3 Guillebaud J (1999) *Contraception: your questions answered* (3e). Churchill Livingstone, London.

4 Scholes D, Stergachis A, Heindrich FE *et al.* (1996) Prevention of pelvic inflammatory disease by screening for cervical chlamydial infection. *NEJM.* **334**: 1362–6.

5 Royal College of Obstetricians and Gynaecologists (1998) *Male and Female Sterilisation*. Royal College of Obstetricians and Gynaecologists, London.

CHAPTER 5

Vaginal discharge, thrush and bacterial vaginosis

Vaginal discharge

It is difficult to know how commonly vaginal discharge causes a problem. Most prevalence studies have looked at specific infections rather than the whole continuum of vaginal discharge complaints. Some vaginal discharge is normal and physiological. The amount and type varies throughout the cycle, from being very scanty just after the menses, through the thin (like egg white) and profuse amount around mid-cycle, to the stage of being thick and easy to roll up into a ball after ovulation. Many complaints about vaginal discharge are due to lack of information about the variations during the cycle, and lack of awareness that increases in amounts can be due to irritation caused by chemicals such as soaps or perfumes, or pressure from clothes or seating. Persistent complaints of discharge in the absence of other symptoms, signs or evidence of infection should make you think about a possible sexual problem or a phobia.

Possible causes

Always take a sexual history. You need to find out whether there is a higher risk of sexually transmitted infection. Referral to the genito-urinary medicine (GUM) clinic for specialised investigations and contact tracing is required if:

- the symptoms started after a recent change of partner, or intercourse with several partners, or an unknown partner
- recurrent or persistent symptoms occur despite simple investigations or treatments
- the partner also has symptoms

- symptoms or signs suggest the involvement of other body systems (e.g. rash, joint pain, generalised enlarged lymph glands).

A list of common and less common causes is given in Box 5.1.

Box 5.1 Causes of vaginal discharge (derived from *Symptom Sorter*[1])

Common	*Less common*	*Rare*
Excess normal secretions	Cervical ectropion	Cancer of the vulva or the vagina
Thrush (monilia, candida)	Cervical polyp	Cervical or uterine cancer
Bacterial vaginosis (BV)	Foreign body (e.g. tampon, ring pessary or other object)	Sloughing uterine fibroid
Trichomonas vaginitis (TV)	Intrauterine contraceptive device	Uterine or tubal infection
Cervicitis due to chlamydia, herpes or gonococcus	Infection in the Bartholin's glands	Pelvic fistula

---

Management

It can be difficult to know how best to determine the cause of the complaint. A busy practice nurse or GP is not going to be able to undertake the detailed investigations that are routine in a GUM clinic. It is sensible to draw up guidelines for the management of vaginal discharge that are practicable within your own working environment. Most patients who complain of a vaginal discharge also have itching and soreness, and most of them will have thrush (candidial vulvovaginitis).[2] Thrush may coexist with other conditions. A suggested approach to basic management is shown in Figure 5.1.

Remember to offer a chaperone for any examination. Just asking if the patient would like someone else with her (a nurse or a friend) will often make her feel more comfortable about the idea of an examination, even if she does not want anyone else present. If you do not examine the patient on the first occasion, give her a definite date by which she should return for further advice if her condition has not improved. An examination can be very helpful in avoiding unnecessary repeated prescriptions for 'thrush' that is not thrush, and for removing a retained tampon at an early stage.

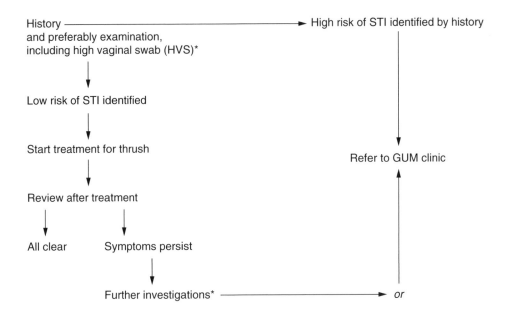

*Investigations performed will depend on the availability of transport and laboratory tests, and on informed consent from the patient for examination.

Figure 5.1: Basic management of the first complaint of vaginal discharge in primary care.

If you are going to perform any investigations, you must explain why you are doing them, what you are looking for, and the implications if an infection other than thrush is found. The patient must be willing to be contacted about the results, or you should document what action she will take to obtain the results if she does not want you to contact her. Remind the patient that you cannot give the results to another person without her written consent. It is surprising how often mothers, partners or friends are asked to pick up the results for patients because they are busy!

Other investigations may be suggested by the history. Health professionals with a special interest might look at the discharge under the microscope themselves – but this is time-consuming in a busy surgery. If the urine test for chlamydia is available in your area, this is an acceptable non-invasive test to add to the routine, especially if there is a reason for suspicion (*see* Chapter 6). Suggested investigations are listed in Table 5.1.

Table 5.1 Suggested investigations for vaginal discharge indicated by the history

Test	Useful for
HVS	*Candida*, bacterial vaginosis, *Trichomonas*
Cervical exudate swab and urethral swab	Gram stain shows Gram-negative diplococcus in about half of all gonococcal infections; culture in addition will detect about 90%[2]
Cervical swab from transitional zone (as for a smear) and/or urethral swab	*Chlamydia trachomatis*
First-catch urine (*not* midstream urine)	DNA amplification tests for *Chlamydia trachomatis*
Specialist investigation	Cancer, upper genital infections, pelvic fistula

Thrush (monilial vulvovaginitis; genital candidiasis)

First or occasional attacks

Most patients and health professionals in primary care are only too familiar with this condition. The first attack may be extremely uncomfortable, with the swelling, itching, soreness and discharge causing considerable distress. Although it is often described as typically presenting with white 'cottage-cheese'-like patches over bright red areas of the vulval or vaginal walls, this presentation is more frequent in pregnancy. The appearance of the discharge may be very variable, and the vulva may be fissured or red and shiny from frequent scratching. Most women complain mainly of the following:

- itching and soreness
- a rapid onset, often in the premenstrual week
- painful urination and/or sexual intercourse.

Guidelines from the British Mycological Society on the management of thrush in general practice appear in the publication *Guidelines*.[3] Topical treatment with an imidazole is usually successful for the first or an occasional attack.

Clotrimazole, econazole, ketoconazole, miconazole and isoconazole are available as cream or pessaries. Treat both the vagina and the vulva. Pessaries for treating the vaginitis are currently more expensive over the counter than a prescription charge in the UK, but the cream is not. Patients may prefer just to have a prescription for the pessaries, and to buy the cream themselves. Short courses are easier to finish. Nystatin pessaries and cream are less effective and require a 14-day course. Oral treatment with fluconazole (one 150 mg tablet) or itraconazole (200 mg repeated once after 8 hours) is popular with patients, especially if the vulva is very inflamed. The oral treatment is contraindicated in pregnancy, is more expensive and does not have a higher cure rate. Treatment with imidazoles (topical and oral) is available over the counter without prescription, but because of the cost you will see many women who have treated only the vulval area.

Recurrent vulvovaginal candidiasis

This is usually defined as 'at least four mycologically proven symptomatic episodes within 12 months'.[4] Only 5% of women with thrush have recurrent candidal vulvovaginitis.

Current research suggests that women who experience recurrent attacks are reacting in the same way to *Candida* as those with hay fever react to pollens – that is, they are producing an allergic reaction to the presence of *Candida* spores and hyphae on the vulval or vaginal mucosa.[4]

Precipitating secondary causes include the following:[4]

- broad-spectrum antibiotics
- pregnancy
- high-dosage combined oral contraceptives (20 or 30 microgram pills are *not* associated with an increased incidence)
- diabetes mellitus
- immune suppression
- genital dermatoses (e.g. eczema or psoriasis)
- nylon or tight-fitting clothes
- hygiene practices such as using soap, Dove, bubble bath, etc., to wash out the vagina
- using antiseptics in the vagina
- sexual intercourse without a condom, which lowers the vaginal pH and causes microfissures.

Clinical presentation can be very variable.

Management should include the following:[4]

- *advice*: that it is not an STI and not a cause of infertility; discuss what precipitates it for that woman, including any cyclical features that could be suppressed (e.g. periods)
- *vulval skin care*: keeping dry and cool; taking showers, not baths; no douching; avoiding perfumes, soap, detergents, antiseptics and deodorants (preparations 'balanced' for the skin are for pH 7.4, not pH 4.6 of the vagina); using aqueous cream instead of soap
- *antifungal therapy*: usually this produces mycological clearance – resistance is very rare; oral treatment is no more effective than local treatment; remember to warn the patient about avoiding pregnancy if using oral therapy
- *recurrent attacks*: may need 3–6 months of continuous or intermittent therapy (depending on the cyclical or precipitating factors); some people need higher doses, as with any medication
- *treating the partner*: this makes no difference to the frequency of attacks, but the ejaculate is alkaline and raises the pH, making thrush more likely to invade. Microfissures in the vulval mucosa that are caused by sexual activity may increase susceptibility to infections of all types.
- *treating the gut*: this makes no difference (and the types of *Candida* in the gut may be different to those in the vagina, so there is *not* a reservoir in the gut)
- *discussion of diets and homeopathy*: there is no good evidence that they work, but reduction of refined sugar and carbohydrates is unlikely to cause harm; exclusion of yeast products may be difficult, and there is no good evidence that it helps; other treatments that patients may ask about are Maritake mushroom supplementation (there is no evidence for its benefits or disadvantages) or *Lactobacillus acidophilus* (one small study from Sweden showed a short-term improvement).[4]

Bacterial vaginosis

Bacterial vaginosis (BV) may be even more common than thrush.[5] It was formerly called *Gardnerella vaginosis*, and is the overgrowth of predominantly anaerobic bacteria that are normally only present in small numbers in the healthy vagina. They produce a fishy or ammonia-like smell in alkaline conditions, so the condition may be worse after intercourse or just after the menses have finished.

BV is of increasing concern to health professionals for the following reasons:

- pelvic inflammatory disease
- endometritis
- post-operative cuff infection after abdominal or vaginal hysterectomy
- post-abortal infection
- psychosexual problems (the smell!)
- obstetric factors (e.g. late miscarriage rates increased, chorioendometritis, pre-term delivery)
- cofactor in HIV transmission.

Management

Tell patients that bacterial vaginosis is a common condition, due to the imbalance of bacteria in the vagina. Advise them that it can resolve spontaneously or recur, and where possible to avoid hygiene practices that disturb the vaginal flora.

Causes of changes in the vaginal flora include the following:

- douching
- antibiotic therapy
- post-partum
- STIs
- foreign body
- menses
- IUD
- post-menopausal
- semen
- malignancy.

Many women improve with simple measures by correcting the alteration of the vaginal flora, particularly by preventing the entry of detergents, soaps and other 'skin-friendly' preparations that are designed to keep the pH at 7.4, rather than at the more acid pH of the vagina.

- *Oral treatment*: metronidazole 2 g as a single dose or 400 mg twice daily for 5–7 days.
- *Vaginal treatment*: metronidazole gel 0.75% for 5 days or clindamycin cream 2% for 7 days (the clindamycin cream can cause condom weakening).

Do not treat the partner. There is no evidence for a 'rectal reservoir' of infection.[6]

Why does treatment fail? The cause may be any of the following:

- lack of compliance with treatment (2 g metronidazole administered as an oral dose has a higher cure rate than longer lower-dose courses)
- other infections
- continuation of hygiene practices that exacerbate the condition.

The relapse rate is 60% in the next three months.

Screening for BV[6]

There is some evidence to suggest that screening after a previous pre-term delivery may be able to prevent a recurrence. Otherwise screening *asymptomatic* women has not been shown to prevent any of the obstetric complications.

- *Screening before IUD insertion*: there is no evidence to support or disprove this at present.
- *Screening and treating before abortion or hysterectomy*: expert opinion suggests that this may be of benefit.
- *Screening before* in-vitro *fertilisation*: the evidence is that bacterial vaginosis does not affect conception rates, but the relative risk (RR) for miscarriage is 2.03 (i.e. there is a doubling of the risk of miscarriage in women with bacterial vaginosis compared with those without BV).[6]

Reflection exercises

Exercise 14

If you do not have guidelines for the management of vaginal discharge, this is a good time to set them up for your practice or clinic. You might want to have a uniform system across all of the sexual health clinics or within a primary care organisation. If you have guidelines already, revise them in the light of recent advances. Look at the guidelines that are available and set up a meeting of the relevant people to discuss and modify them as necessary. You might want to involve all of the clinical staff involved in managing vaginal discharge, or ask for representatives if there are large numbers of staff. You might want to seek expert advice on particular aspects (e.g. what tests are available, and their sensitivity and specificity) from a bacteriologist and/or a GUM specialist. Would it be useful to have the guidelines readily available (e.g. as a template on the computer, or as a laminated A4 sheet, or in a folder)?

Exercise 15

You may want to draw up protocols so that the practice nurses and district nurses are able to take over the investigation and management of vaginal discharge. Are they all feeling confident about how to take swabs and what swabs to take? Set up a meeting with an expert (perhaps one of the GUM nurses) to go through the protocol and discuss any procedures.

Exercise 16

Do you know what type of service your patients would prefer? To find out, you could ask a representative group or groups, hold focus group meetings, or design a questionnaire. You might ask who they would prefer to consult – for example, which of the following options they would prefer:

- a nurse or doctor
- a male or female health professional
- go directly to a GUM clinic
- go to a combined contraceptive and sexual healthcare clinic.

Collate the answers and feed back the findings to your practice team meeting, your primary care organisation, clinical lead or trust management for action.

Now that you have completed one or more of the interactive reflection exercises in this chapter, transfer the information from this needs assessment to the empty templates. Use the personal development plan on pages 148–158 if you are working on your own learning plan, or the practice or workplace personal and professional development plan on pages 174–181 if you are working on a practice or workplace team learning plan. The conclusions reached at the end of each exercise will feature in the action plan. Don't forget to keep the evidence of your learning in your personal portfolio.

References

1 Hopcroft K and Forte V (1999) *Symptom Sorter*. Radcliffe Medical Press, Oxford.

2 Adler MW (1988) *ABC of Sexually Transmitted Diseases*. BMJ Books, London.

3 Foord-Kelcey G (ed.) (2001) *Guidelines. Volume 13*. Medendium Group Publishing Ltd, Berkhamsted.

4 Ringdahl EN (2000) Treatment of recurrent vulvovaginal candidiasis (review). *Am Fam Physician*. **61**: 3306–12, 3317.

5 Sonnex C (1996) *A General Practitioner's Guide to Genitourinary Medicine and Sexual Health*. Cambridge University Press, Cambridge.

6 Barton S (2001) *Clinical Evidence. Issue 5*. BMJ Publishing Group, London.

CHAPTER 6

Chlamydia trachomatis

Introduction

You may wish to include proposals for implementing screening for chlamydial infection in your personal or practice development plan.[1]

Chlamydial infection is frequently asymptomatic, but is a common cause of infertility and chronic pelvic infection.[2] It is a frequent cause of ectopic pregnancy and chronic pelvic pain. Ascending infection in men causes epididymitis, but evidence of male infertility is limited. Maternal-to-infant transmission causes neonatal conjunctivitis and pneumonitis. It may coexist with other STIs, and may contribute to the transmission and acquisition of HIV infection.

A randomised controlled trial involving the screening of asymptomatic women regarded as 'high risk' found a clinically significant reduction in the incidence of pelvic inflammatory disease in the intervention group.[3] Observational data from Sweden[4] and the USA[5] support the effectiveness of screening for chlamydial infection.

Nucleic acid amplification tests have been developed that are highly sensitive (over 90%) compared with the standard endocervical enzyme immunoassay (EIA) test (which has a lower sensitivity of 60–70%). Reports of the use of nucleic acid amplification testing on urine samples in primary care are being published.[6,7] The urine samples need to be the first passed fraction of the urine, not midstream samples, in order to collect the organisms from the urethra.

Introducing screening requires a knowledge of how the diagnosis is made and how the condition is treated.[8] A higher index of suspicion and greater patient demand for testing is likely to follow the growing publicity about chlamydia. There are already concerns about the ability of health services to shoulder the burden of previously undetected disease, and the follow-up of infections will pose many problems for those health professionals who are insufficiently informed or skilled.[9,10] Informed consent about screening for a sexually transmitted infection cannot be obtained without a discussion of sexuality and sexual health.

Many health professionals feel less than competent in this area, and have received little undergraduate or postgraduate training in sexual health.[11]

Screening

If you initiate screening procedures, you should have conclusive evidence that screening can alter the natural history of that disease in a significant proportion of those individuals who are screened.[12] You might think about the factors listed in Box 6.1.

Box 6.1 General principles to consider when introducing screening of asymptomatic people for illnesses or infections with special reference to chlamydia

Is the condition important?	Chlamydia is an important cause of infertility, ectopic pregnancy, salpingitis, chronic pelvic pain and morbidity
Is the natural history well understood?	Around 70–80% of women have cervical infections with no symptoms, but it is not clear how many have a risk of ascending infections in the absence of precipitating factors, such as instrumentation of the uterus
Is there a recognisable early stage?	Screening tests can identify asymptomatic infection
Is there a suitable test?	The nucleic acid amplification tests are more sensitive and specific than the previous EIA tests
Is the test acceptable?	Urine tests are more acceptable than cervical or urethral swabs
At what intervals should the test be repeated?	Unknown – and may depend on the accuracy and completeness of contact tracing and treatment, and on social factors such as change of partner or monogamy

---

Are there adequate facilities for diagnosis and treatment?	No – primary care health professionals do not have sufficient time or skills, GUM clinics could not cope with the number of referrals of people with positive tests, and the laboratories have insufficient capacity and resources to perform the tests
Is treatment at an early stage of more benefit than treatment at a later stage?	Definitely – infection can easily be eradicated in the early stages before structural damage occurs
Is the likelihood of physical and psychological harm less than the likelihood of benefit?	This depends on how the test is presented, people's feelings about stigmatisation (having a 'sexually transmitted infection') and public knowledge about the condition
Can the cost be balanced against the benefits that the service provides, versus other opportunity costs and benefits?	Unknown as yet – pilot studies from Merseyside[13] and Southampton showed a much higher prevalence of infection and higher costs for the counselling time and number of tests performed than expected

Who might you test?

You might wish to draw up your own guidelines for identifying infection based on others already available (e.g. the Royal College of Physicians guidelines[14] or the SIGN guidelines[15]).

You must always consider the implications of screening and be prepared to explain to the patient exactly what is involved and the implications if they do have a positive result. There is no point in screening if you cannot contact the person with the results (positive and negative), or if he or she then refuses treatment for a positive result.

The guidelines mentioned above suggest that you might target the following asymptomatic women for opportunistic screening:

- those who are under the age of 25 years
- those who have had a recent change of partner or more than two partners in the last year

- those who do not use barrier contraception
- those with a higher risk of STIs because of their lifestyle.

You should also consider screening symptomatic patients:

- women with vaginal discharge, post-coital or intermenstrual bleeding, an inflamed cervix (that may bleed on contact), urethritis, pelvic inflammatory disease and lower abdominal pain or reactive arthritis in the sexually active
- women undergoing uterine instrumentation (e.g. termination of pregnancy, intrauterine contraceptive device insertion), sexual partners of those with suspected infection or other STIs, and mothers of infants with chlamydial conjunctivitis
- men with urethral discharge, dysuria or urethritis, as well as epididymitis or reactive arthritis in the sexually active.

Box 6.2

H attended for emergency contraception. On taking a history, the nurse discovered that unprotected intercourse had taken place several times in the last week since the day that the patient's last period finished, and that this was a new relationship, the previous one having ended two months previously when H had stopped taking the pill. The nurse referred H to the doctor who, after obtaining informed consent, took swabs from the cervix and vagina. Erring on the side of caution, the doctor gave H an immediate dose of azithromycin,[16] and, as she was within the time limits for emergency contraception, fitted an intrauterine contraceptive device.

What test should be used?

The recommended test for chlamydia according to the SIGN guidelines[15] is the nucleic acid amplification test, but this may need to be modified according to the availability of the test in your area. Testing the urine (the whole specimen, not midstream urine) is much more acceptable than a urethral or cervical swab, especially if a genital examination is not indicated for other reasons. Enzyme immunoassay or immunofluorescence tests may be the only ones available, but they are less specific and sensitive. A cervical swab should be taken from the transitional zone (as for a cervical smear) after cleaning off excess mucus with cotton wool. Taking a urethral swab as well as a cervical swab in women increases the likelihood of identifying chlamydia. Use swabs with plastic shafts as wooden shafts are toxic to chlamydia. The decision as to whether to rate swabs from other sites (e.g. the rectum or oropharynx) in either men or women will depend on the sexual history obtained.

What treatment should be given?

The recommendations for women undergoing termination of pregnancy[17,18] suggest that all such patients should be given antibiotic treatment to eradicate chlamydia. However, this ignores the cardinal rules of treatment for STIs – that is, diagnose first and treat all of the contacts. If possible, swabs to identify chlamydia (as suggested above) should be taken before treatment is given, but treatment should be given before the termination of pregnancy even if the result is not yet available. A positive chlamydia result should result in partner notification and treatment, preferably by the GUM clinic, although this is not always easy to do.[18]

A useful summary of effective treatments appears in *Clinical Evidence*,[19] on which the information in Box 6.3 is based.

Box 6.3 Treatment of chlamydia

Uncomplicated genital infection in men and non-pregnant women	Good evidence for effectiveness of oral treatment: • azithromycin, 1 g single dose • doxycycline, 100 mg twice daily for 7 days • oxytetracycline, 250 mg four times daily for 7 days. Uncertain evidence for effectiveness of treatment: • ofloxacin, 200 mg twice daily for 7 days • minocycline, 100 mg once daily for 9 days • lymecycline, 300 mg once daily for 10 days Unlikely to work as a treatment: • ciprofloxacin multiple doses

Uncomplicated infection in pregnancy	Good evidence for effectiveness of treatment:
	• azithromycin, 1 g single dose
	• erythromycin, 500 mg four times daily for 7 days
	• amoxycillin, 500 mg three times daily for 7 days.
	Uncertain evidence for effectiveness of treatment:
	• clindamycin.

You are likely to need to refer men or women with upper genital tract or disseminated infection for specialist management. Men with epididymitis, women with pelvic inflammatory disease, and individuals of either sex with perihepatitis or reactive arthritis often require specialist investigation. Box 6.4 lists some treatment schedules for upper genital tract infections, but you are likely to be advised on this by the clinician in secondary care.

Box 6.4 Treatment of upper or disseminated genital tract infection

In men   Doxycycline, 100 mg twice daily for 7 to 14 days.
            Oxytetracycline, 250 mg four times daily for 7 to 14 days.

In women   As other organisms are usually present, treatment is usually combined with metronidazole 400 mg twice daily for 7 days, or with clindamycin 450 mg four times daily.
            Doxycycline, 100 mg for 10 to 14 days, or
            Ofloxacin, 400 mg twice a day.

If symptoms and signs of infection are present, you may decide to start treatment immediately without waiting for confirmation from laboratory testing.

Partner tracing and treatment

For every person with a positive test there are at least two other infected individuals. Ideally, patients should be referred to the GUM clinic where trained health advisers can undertake the contact tracing and arrange for treatment. No one method of contact tracing or partner notification has been shown to be more effective than another, but telephone reminders and contact cards have been found to be helpful.[7] If you cannot persuade individuals to attend GUM clinics, you should obtain consent and offer the following choice with regard to notification of contacts:

- patient referral – index patients themselves notify their sexual contacts to advise them to seek treatment
- provider referral – the healthcare professional informs the sexual contacts anonymously that they should seek treatment
- conditional referral – the healthcare professional notifies the contact directly if the patient has not managed to do so after a specified number of days.

Usually the sexual contacts who are notified are:

- patients with symptoms – all sexual partners in the last four weeks
- patients without symptoms – all sexual partners in the last six months, or the most recent partner if there has been none for more than six months.

It is not always easy to motivate people to take the risks to their health seriously when the condition may have no symptoms.

Box 6.5

A 17-year-old single parent attended a contraception clinic complaining of post-coital bleeding. Several months previously she had experienced a discharge and painful intercourse, and swabs had shown a positive chlamydia result. She had been referred to the GUM clinic at the time, but had only attended once (she said it was too far to travel). The doctor explained that her symptoms could be due to chlamydia again and enquired about contact tracing. The girl had told her (by then) ex-partner, but he had refused to go for treatment, saying that it was her problem. Although they had split up, she had continued to have intermittent intercourse with him. Now she had a new partner who was complaining of dysuria, and she wanted him to be seen as well! She seemed unconcerned that she had put herself and her new partner at risk by continuing to have sexual contact with the father of her child – and the doctor felt irritated, but also uneasy, that the father of her child seemed to be behaving in an abusive and irresponsible way.

Follow-up

If there is no risk of reinfection, then no test of cure is usually performed. If such a test is required, postpone it until at least three weeks after therapy, otherwise you may obtain false-positive results.

Reflection exercises

Exercise 17

You could arrange for an expert on chlamydia to give a talk to your practice team, or a group of practices in your primary care organsiation, or your clinic staff, to increase the level of knowledge about the condition, the tests available and the treatment. Alternatively, you could attend a course elsewhere and then disseminate your knowledge, supplemented by reading, to others in your practice, primary care organisation, or clinics.

Exercise 18

Conduct a significant event audit of three patients with a recent diagnosis of pelvic inflammatory disease. Establish whether there are any factors that could have altered the development of the condition. Read up about the risk factors for pelvic inflammatory disease, and consider what procedures might help to identify patients at risk and increase the possibility of screening and/or early treatment. Present your findings at a meeting for colleagues and staff.

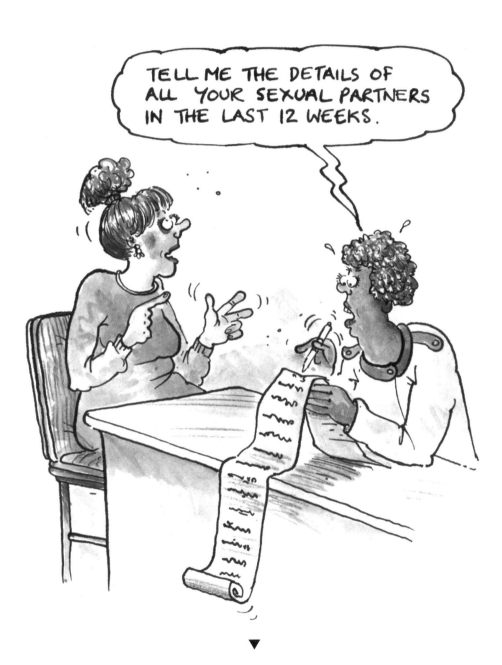

Exercise 19

Find out what screening is performed prior to termination of pregnancy. Does your local provider have a protocol for identifying chlamydia? Are the women treated before the procedure, or do swab results take so long that they are received too late for this?[20] What arrangements are made for follow-up and contact tracing if the swabs are positive? Is the referring doctor notified about the result? When you have found out what happens, you may wish to renegotiate the contract or arrange for cervical swabs to be taken at an earlier stage. You may need to discuss your findings with your primary care organisation, management group, health authority or public health consultant.

> Now that you have completed one or more of the interactive reflection exercises in this chapter, transfer the information from this needs assessment to the empty templates. Use the personal development plan on pages 148–158 if you are working on your own learning plan, or the practice or workplace personal and professional development plan on pages 174–181 if you are working on a practice or workplace team learning plan. The conclusions reached at the end of each exercise will feature in the action plan. Don't forget to keep the evidence of your learning in your personal portfolio.

References

1 Boag F and Kelly F (1998) Screening for *Chlamydia trachomatis*. *BMJ*. **316**: 1474.

2 Lindsay DT, Trouson AO and Anderson AN (1994) Female infertility: causes and treatment. *Lancet*. **343**: 1539–44.

3 Scholes D, Stergachis A, Heidrich FE *et al.* (1996) Prevention of pelvic inflammatory disease by screening for cervical *Chlamydia* infection. *NEJM*. **334**: 1362–6.

4 Egger M, Low N, Davey Smith G *et al.* (1998) Screening for chlamydial infections and the risk of ectopic pregnancies in a county in Sweden: ecological analysis. *BMJ*. **316**: 1776–80.

5 Hillis S, Black C, Newhall J *et al.* (1995) New opportunities for chlamydia prevention: applications of science to public health practice. *Sex Trans Dis*. **22**: 197–210.

6 Grun L, Tassano-Smith J, Carder C *et al.* (1997) Comparison of two methods of screening for genital chlamydial infection in women attending in general practice: cross-sectional survey. *BMJ.* **315**: 226–30.

7 Ostergaard I, Moller JK, Anderson B and Olesen F (1996) Diagnosis of urogenital *Chlamydia trachomatis* infection in women, based on mailed samples obtained at home: multipractice comparative study. *BMJ.* **313**: 1186–9.

8 Southgate L (1990) The diagnosis and management of chlamydial cervicitis: a test of cure. *J Fam Pract.* **31**: 33–5.

9 Southgate L, Treharne J and Williams R (1989) Detection, treatment and follow-up of women with *Chlamydia trachomatis* infection seeking abortion in inner-city general practices. *BMJ.* **299**: 1136–7.

10 Stokes T, Bhaduri S, Schober P and Shukla R (1997) General practitioners' management of genital chlamydia: a survey of reported practice. *Fam Pract.* **14**: 455–60.

11 Wakley G (2000) Sexual health in the primary care consultation: using self-rating as an aid to identifying training needs for general practitioners. *Sex Relation Ther.* **15**: 171–81.

12 Cochrane AL and Holland WW (1971) Validation of screening procedures. *Br Med Bull.* **27**: 3–8.

13 Harvey J, Webb A and Mallinson H (2000) *Chlamydia trachomatis* screening in young people in Merseyside. *Br J Fam Plan.* **26**: 199–201.

14 Foord-Kelcey G (ed.) (2001) *Guidelines, Volume 13.* Medendium Group Publishing Ltd, Berkhamsted.

15 Scottish Intercollegiate Guidelines Network (SIGN) (2000) *Management of genital Chlamydia trachomatis Infection.* SIGN, Edinburgh.

16 Grimes DA and Schulzt KF (2001) Antibiotic prophylaxis for intrauterine contraceptive device insertion (Cochrane Review). In: *The Cochrane Library. Issue 1.* Update Software, Oxford.

17 Penney GC, Thomson M, Norman J *et al.* (1998) A randomised comparison of strategies for reducing infective complications of induced abortion. *Br J Obstet Gynaecol.* **105**: 599–604.

18 Royal College of Obstetricians and Gynaecologists (2000) *Guidelines for Induced Abortion.* Royal College of Obstetricians and Gynaecologists, London.

19 Barton S (2001) *Clinical Evidence. Issue 5.* BMJ Publishing Group, London.

20 Smith CD, Liu DTY, Jushuf IA and Hammond RH (2001) Genital infection and termination of pregnancy: are patients still at risk? *Br J Fam Plan Reprod Health Care.* **27**: 81–4.

CHAPTER 7

Sexually transmitted infections (STIs)

Introduction

The number of people with sexually transmitted infections (STIs) has been increasing overall from 1990 to 1999.[1] Genitourinary medicine (GUM) clinics are responsible for making statistical returns to the Department of Health of the number of cases of STIs seen each year, categorised by diagnosis and gender. The latest statistics from the Public Health Laboratory Service always lag behind what is currently detected in practice. Moreover, the STI rates from GUM clinics will always be an underestimate, as some cases will be treated in general practice or by other hospital departments (e.g. gynaecology departments), but they are the nearest we can get to assessing what is happening in sexual health. The number of new diagnoses and the uptake of services in GUM clinics exceeded one million for the first time in 1998 – infection rates that were 6% higher than in 1997.[1]

The Department of Health selected gonorrhoea as a marker of sexual practices in *The Health of the Nation*[2] targets (the target being to reduce the incidence of gonorrhoea by 20% by the year 2000).

The number of gonorrhoea cases increased between 1997 and 1998, with the largest rises occurring in London, and preliminary data indicate even bigger rises between 1998 and 1999. Those aged between 16 and 19 years were particularly affected, with increases of up to 52% in males and 39% in females in this age group.

The rate of identification of chlamydial infections is rising everywhere. This may be partly due to greater awareness of the significance of chlamydial infection. The number of chlamydia infections in men increased by 17% and in women by 11% between 1997 and 1998. Chlamydial infections are particularly likely to occur in young people under the age of 20 years.

The steepest rise in the number of first attacks of genital warts was in young men and women aged 16–19 years, and overall the rate increased by 2% between 1997 and 1998. Herpes simplex virus infections also increased, but mainly in those over 45 years of age. It is difficult to know whether STI rates are continuing to rise, whether people are more prepared to attend GUM clinics, or whether health professionals are more aware of the possibility of STIs.

What you can tell people about genitourinary medicine (GUM) clinics[3]

The new name for these clinics causes some confusion. They were previously known as 'special' or 'VD' (venereal disease) clinics, or sometimes 'STD' (sexually transmitted disease) clinics – as well as by many nicknames, such as the 'clap clinic', the 'back-lane' clinic, etc. Access to these clinics varies across the country, and new users often find it difficult to find out what is available. Healthcare workers should know where these clinics are located and how people can be seen. Some clinics have open access, while others require appointments to be made by telephone. Some are open in the evening, while others are only open from 10 a.m. to 5 p.m. (not very convenient!). Some of the clinics now have a seamless one-stop service together with contraceptive clinics, or are on the same premises to allow easy transfers between the services. Others only provide contraception in emergencies.

It needs to be emphasised that the service is confidential and that the records are kept separately from other hospital records. By law, staff in a GUM clinic cannot tell a patient what infection their partner has, or tell their doctor that they have attended, unless the patient requests this. The clinic cannot give any information to other doctors, solicitors, insurance companies or the police without the patient's consent. The clinic will record a name and a date of birth, and will ask for a contact address so that results can be given (but patients do not have to give this information if they prefer not to).

After taking a detailed history, often using a check-list, tests can be performed immediately to diagnose some infections. For other tests it will take some time before the results are known. The clinic does need some identifying information so that they can access patients' records when they reattend. All treatment is provided free of charge.

Cervical smears can also be taken, and some clinics can examine the cervix for abnormalities with a colposcope. Some GUM clinics will have sexual problem counsellors or impotence clinics attached to them. All of them have health advisers who can discuss sexual health with clients openly and honestly.

GUM clinics try hard to be effective in tracing sexual contacts when an infection is present. They may give clients a slip of paper with a coded diagnosis to give to partners or ex-partners, who can then take the slip to *any* GUM clinic and be tested and treated. If clients prefer, the health adviser can contact partners to tell them that they may have been exposed to infection.

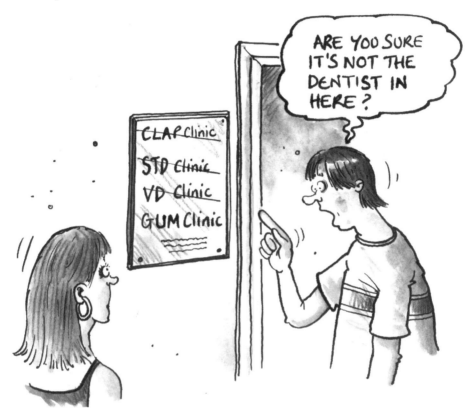

Presentation of sexually transmitted infections (STIs)

Patients may present at their general practice or at a clinic with any of the following:

- irritation
- painful urination
- discharge from the urethra or vagina
- lumps on the genital area or elsewhere
- ulcers

- pain in the genital area
- information or a suspicion that their partner has an STI.

Suspicion about the presence of STIs may be raised by finding any of the following:

- a raised number of white blood cells (WBC) with no organisms cultured from the urine
- pelvic pain or dyspareunia
- perihepatitis or periappendicitis
- menstrual irregularities or intermenstrual bleeding
- cervical smear abnormalities
- miscarriage
- ectopic pregnancy
- premature labour
- conjunctivitis
- reactive arthritis.

The main point is to remember to think about the possibility of STIs! Everyone who has had sexual contact with a partner is at risk, unless they have both only ever had contact with each other. Monogamous monogamy or chastity provide the only (almost) complete protection. The other risks are from non-sexual exchange of body fluids, such as needlestick injuries, sharing injection needles, or transmission from mother to infant, but not from toilet seats.

Bacterial vaginosis was discussed in Chapter 5 and chlamydial infection was described in Chapter 6. Other causes of discharge, and additional aspects of sexually transmitted infections that are commonly encountered in primary care, are discussed in this chapter. The Clinical Effectiveness Group of the Association for Genitourinary Medicine and the Medical Society for the Study of Venereal Diseases have produced national guidelines for the management of STIs, which are freely available on their website.[4]

Trichomonas vaginalis

This flagellate organism occurs in the urethra in both sexes, but also in the vagina and paraurethral glands in women. In adults it is the cause of a sexually transmitted disease and is frequently associated with other STIs. Babies can acquire the infection perinatally from an infected mother, but after that age a proven infection would provoke investigations of sexual abuse.

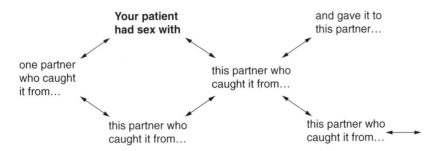

Figure 7.1: Contacts of infection.

The commonest complaint in both men and women is of discharge, but 15–50% of men have no symptoms.[4] Women also complain of itching, dysuria or a smelly discharge. Although the discharge is classically described as having a frothy yellow appearance, it is often variable in both consistency and colour.

Diagnosis in primary care is usually made from the culture of a high vaginal swab taken into a suitable transport medium. For male patients, send a urethral swab or first-pass urine sample (preferably both) for culture. In women, beware of making the diagnosis from a cervical smear. The false-positive rate of 30% may cause psychological harm and unwarranted accusations of partner unfaithfulness if a patient whose diagnosis was made solely on the basis of a cervical smear result is referred or treated without confirmation of the diagnosis by culture.[4]

Treat sexual partners simultaneously if possible, and advise abstinence from sexual intercourse until treatment of *all* partners is completed. (Condom use reduces the transmission of STIs,[5] but abstinence is better.) In addition, screening for other STIs must be arranged. Contact tracing is also needed – remember that there are at least two other individuals to be treated apart from the person you have seen (*see* Figure 7.1). Preferably arrange screening and contact tracing by referral to the GUM clinic.

Treatment is with oral metronidazole, either 2 g as a single dose (this has better compliance and is cheaper) or 400 mg twice daily for 5–7 days (there is some evidence that this has a higher cure rate). Use of the lower dose for a longer time is recommended in pregnancy.[6] Remember to give advice about avoiding alcohol while taking metronidazole. There is only about a 5% failure rate with metronidazole if the drug is taken correctly – most failures are due to not taking it or to reinfection. Test of cure is normally only performed if symptoms persist.

Box 7.1

Ms M, a manager, was dressed in a suit and held her briefcase like a shield on her lap before carefully putting it on the floor. She hesitated and then said that she had to sort it out. She told the doctor that she had had a phone call from a colleague who accused her of giving him 'the clap'. Looking away from the doctor's gaze, she recounted that she had spent the night with him while at a meeting – she knew he was married but they had spent the night together on several occasions previously. She had nothing wrong with her, she was sure, but he had insisted that he had started with a discharge after sleeping with her and now she wanted a check-up to make sure she had not caught anything. She had no complaints, no discharge, no dysuria and no abdominal pain. The doctor suggested a full screening at the GUM clinic, but she insisted that she could not go there. They compromised by arranging delivery of the swabs to the laboratory that afternoon and used a suitable pseudonym with the surgery address to ensure anonymity of the results. Unfortunately for Ms M, she did have to make the time to attend a GUM clinic (she attended one outside her management area), as gonococcus was isolated from the cervical and urethral swabs.

Gonorrhoea

The incidence of this infection is increasing, especially among 16 to 19-year-olds.[7] Infection can be asymptomatic in about 10% of men and 50% of women. Male symptoms of dysuria, discharge or epididymitis, or female symptoms of discharge, dysuria or abdominal pain should raise your suspicions. The goncoccocus infects mucous membranes, so swabs need to be taken from the urethra or the endocervix. Other sites (pharyngeal or rectal swabs) may be indicated by the history (highlighting the importance of taking a good sexual history). Referral to a GUM clinic for full STI screening, contact tracing and advice on current antibiotic sensitivities is best practice. It is essential that female contacts are traced and treated, as long-term adverse effects of pelvic infection can occur even in asymptomatic patients.

Non-specific urethritis or non-specific genital infection

This is defined as an infection, usually urethritis, that is not caused by gonorrhoea. It is common in young men. Up to 40% of episodes of urethritis are in fact caused by chlamydia. *Mycoplasma genitalium* and *Ureaplasma urealyticum* are the commonest of the other causative organisms. The diagnosis is mainly made on the basis of a combination of symptoms of urethritis and the presence of pus cells – more than five per high-power field ($\times 400$) – from a urethral swab. The partner(s) should be treated to prevent recurrence. Treatment is the same as for chlamydia.

Genital warts – human papilloma virus (HPV)

The incidence of first-ever presentation of genital warts is rising, again with a significant increase in the 16–19 years age group.[1] HPV infection is common among sexually active young people whether or not visible warts are present. Genital warts are usually spread sexually, so their presence should prompt a search for other STIs. Some HPVs (types 16, 18, 31, 33 and 35)[1] – not usually the ones presenting as visible warts – are associated with the development of cervical cancer, and yearly cervical screening for five years is normally suggested if wart virus is found. Determination of the type of HPV present is still a research technique at the time of writing. Investigations are under way to determine the feasibility of using it to distinguish between those individuals who require more frequent follow-up and those whose infection is likely to be transient and not associated with a greater risk of cervical cancer.

Treatment is usually started with podophyllin. This is very irritating and should be washed off three to four hours after its application. It is not suitable for self-application, as patients often overtreat themselves in the hope of obtaining a speedy cure, and can experience nasty burns, or even peripheral neuropathy, hypokalaemia or coma, after applying large quantities. Podophyllotoxin 0.5% has less severe side-effects and can be applied by patients at home if they can localise the warts accurately (this is easier with penile warts than with those in other positions!) Trichloracetic acid, electrocautery or cryotherapy are also used for larger or more resistant warts. *Clinical Evidence* states that the researchers found no clear evidence of the superiority of one treatment over another.[5] Podophyllotoxin, imiquimod and intralesional interferon were all found to be more effective than placebo, but other treatments had not been adequately evaluated. The effects of treatment are difficult to assess because of natural regression (about 30% of cases) and also recurrences after treatment. Furthermore, *Clinical Evidence* reports no evidence that treatment of external warts reduces infectivity, and reported that the preventive effects of condom use had not been adequately evaluated.

Herpes simplex

Although they are less significant than other STIs in terms of numbers, herpes infections cause severe morbidity. The first attack is often extremely painful, sometimes causing retention of urine because of the severe pain as urine passes over the lesions. Recurrent attacks prevent sexual enjoyment and may permanently adversely affect the quality of life, especially if recurrences are frequent. *Clinical Evidence* found that oral antiviral treatment reduced the duration of symptoms, lesions and viral shedding. Research reported that daily treatment reduced recurrences and may improve the quality of life. There was limited evidence that condom use reduced the rate of transmission.[5]

Giving advice to pregnant women who have recurrent herpes is difficult. An abdominal delivery reduces the likelihood of transmission to the baby, but with greater risks of maternal morbidity and mortality. The highest risk of transmission to the baby is in women with a first infection in late pregnancy, and there is limited evidence that antiviral treatment reduces the number of women with recurrent disease who have genital lesions at term.

Syphilis

New cases of syphilis in the UK are uncommon, and are mostly found by screening in pregnancy or for blood donation. The presence of a solitary ulcer or the rash of secondary syphilis may raise suspicions. Referral to a GUM clinic is essential.

Viral hepatitis

Several different virus types cause hepatitis, all of which can cause an acute illness with jaundice. Asymptomatic infections are common. Hepatitis B and D also cause chronic infection progressing to cirrhosis and liver failure. Hepatitis B is more infectious than human immunodeficiency virus (HIV), and can be spread by sexual intercourse as well as via contaminated blood. Hepatitis A can be caught sexually from a partner with an active infection. Immunisation against hepatitis A is now available, either separately or together with hepatitis B immunisation, and should be considered for at-risk groups and travellers.

Human immunodeficiency virus (HIV) and acquired immunodeficiency syndrome (AIDS)

New presentations of symptomatic HIV and AIDS diagnoses in homosexual men fell by 45% between 1997 and 1998. The number of new HIV infections has risen overall, and they are now commoner in people who have *heterosexual* intercourse than in those who have homosexual intercourse.[8] The increase in other STIs suggests that the safe-sex message is being forgotten in both homosexual and heterosexual relationships. The long-term implications of a diagnosis if no symptoms are present have to be considered carefully before a test is performed. The health advisers at GUM clinics are experienced in explaining the risk–benefit ratio to people who think that they may have been exposed to risk. If you are to give people good advice both about their risks and about the implications of testing, ensure that you are up to date and accurate. Counselling is ideally undertaken within primary care, but has implications for workload (it is time consuming), training and education (it is a rapidly changing field) and confidentiality (many patients do not feel confident about the standards of confidentiality in primary care). In areas with low rates of infection, referral to a central clinic is probably preferable, but health professionals in areas of higher incidence should consider their learning needs, what expertise they require and what provision is needed.

The symptoms of an acute infection with HIV may resemble glandular fever, but most cases are asymptomatic. The development of antibodies takes about two to six weeks, but can be longer than this.

Chronic infection may also be asymptomatic, but about one-third of patients have generalised persistently enlarged lymph nodes. Later in the course of the chronic infection, symptoms of night sweats, fever, diarrhoea and weight loss occur. Frequent infections of mucous membranes or skin are often present. About 75% of HIV-positive people develop symptoms over a period of 9–10 years without therapy.[3] As the management of this disease is changing very rapidly, the role of the primary care team is likely to be supportive of the local secondary care management. You need to be aware of the support systems and organisations available, and know where to obtain local expertise.

Pubic lice

This infestation commonly coexists with STIs and is usually sexually acquired, so consider full screening. Treatment is with malathion 0.5%, gammabenzene hexachloride as powder, cream or lotion, or cabaryl 0.5%. It is left in contact with all of the hairy areas except the scalp for 24 hours, and can then be washed off. The patient should wash their clothes and bedclothes in hot water at that time, or have them dry-cleaned. All sexual and family contacts should be treated.

Giving advice about 'safer sex'

Many people have sexually transmitted infections without realising it, and they cannot be identified in advance. The major risk to avoid that has been widely publicised is from HIV infections. However, many people do not know about the other STIs that they are more likely to catch. A needlestick injury gives a 0.3% risk of contracting HIV if it is present, but a 30% risk of catching hepatitis B. Chlamydial and, to a lesser extent, gonococcal infections are all too common among people who change their partner frequently, particularly the young and the newly divorced or separated.

Box 7.2 below summarises the risks associated with various activities.

Box 7.2 The safest sex is with your monogamous partner

High risk — Vaginal or anal intercourse without a condom, including withdrawal (coitus interruptus)
Giving oral sex to a man and allowing the ejaculate into the mouth

Giving oral sex to a woman during her period (menstruation)

Unprotected 'rimming' (licking one's partner's anal area)

Finger insertion with cuts or grazes or during menstruation

Getting human faeces or urine in one's mouth

Sharing sex toys

Unprotected sex with more than one partner after another, or without a change of condom

Medium risk	Vaginal or oral sex with a condom
	Giving oral sex to a man, but not taking the ejaculate into the mouth
	Giving oral sex to a woman during her period, but using protection between oneself and the body fluids
	Giving oral sex to a woman, but not during her period
	'Rimming' with the protection of a barrier (e.g. dental dam*)
	'Wet' kissing (French kissing) with open mouths – this depends on the health of one's lips and mouth. Bleeding gums or ulcers, cut lips, cold sores, etc., increase the risk
	Sharing sex toys after washing (remove the batteries first) and covering them with a fresh condom for each user
	Using a sex toy in the vagina after using it in the anus, and covering it with a fresh condom for each use.
Low or no risk	Masturbation on one's own or with a partner (but make sure that any cuts or grazes are covered by a waterproof plaster, or wear latex gloves)
	Use of personal sex toys (but make sure that they are washed after each use in warm soapy water)
	Kissing on the lips with no exchange of saliva, or kissing on the body
	Hugging, cuddling, body rubbing, sexual arousal when fully clothed, licking food off each other, or other activities that do not involve exchange of body fluids

> Sensual body massage (but ensure that oils do not come into contact with latex or rubber, which they can weaken)
>
> Erotic fantasy, either alone or shared
>
> Anything else that gives mutual pleasure by consent and that does not involve exchange of body fluids
>
> ---
>
> * Dental dams are sheets of latex (rubber) that are used as a protection for oral sex. Place them over the whole of the area beforehand. They can fall off, so mark which side is yours, or it will defeat the object of protection if you replace it the wrong side out! You can also use a flavoured condom by splitting it up the long side to make a barrier.

Too much emphasis on the risks of STIs can be counter-productive. Individuals in the younger age groups in particular often feel (perhaps rightly) that health professionals or other adults are making a 'mountain out of a molehill' in order to control people's sexuality. Factual straightforward information about the risks is all that is needed. Exaggeration or emotive language merely stops people from listening. That is not to say that all the risks of sexual contact, including an unwanted pregnancy, should not be discussed, but this should be done in the context of how enjoyable the activity can be as well!

Bear in mind that Peter Greenhouse defined sexual health as the 'enjoyment of the sexual activity of one's choice without causing or experiencing physical or emotional harm'.[9]

Emphasising the downside of sexual activity can be just as harmful as a person receiving too little information to keep them safe.

Reflection exercises

Exercise 20

One member of the practice or clinic team could be responsible for the supply of up-to-date leaflets on STIs, but all members of the team need to know that they exist, where to find them and what they contain. The responsible member of staff could keep a looseleaf file of relevant leaflets in the common-room or practice library. He or she could arrange a meeting with the health education department, health visitors and school nurses to discuss what health education needs with regard to STIs might be met by the practice or clinic.

Exercise 21

Audit what leaflets are available, and in what location, on a regular basis to ensure their availability. This can be simply done by using a spreadsheet in Excel, listing all of the leaflets and their location, and setting a minimum number that should be available (e.g. five leaflets). If you do not know how to set up a spreadsheet, you have identified yet another learning need – or a job to be delegated to someone who does know how to do it!

Exercise 22

Do your patients feel able to help themselves to leaflets? Would the leaflets be better placed elsewhere (e.g. not in the waiting-room but in a corridor so that it is easier to pick one up unobserved)? You could ask your patient representative group (do you have one yet?) or use a snapshot anonymous questionnaire[10] given to patients in the waiting-room over a couple of weeks.

Exercise 23

Does everyone in the practice/clinic know where and how to refer people to GUM clinics or how people can attend without letting you know? Ask your colleagues informally about this at coffee and tea breaks. If you find gaps in their knowledge, arrange for a speaker from the GUM service to talk to the practice or several practices, or ask the staff of GUM clinics about what services are available and how they can be accessed. You might visit a GUM clinic (out of hours to avoid breaches of confidentiality) so that you can direct patients to the clinic more confidently and give them a first-hand account of what their visit will entail.

Now that you have completed these interactive reflection exercises, transfer the information to the relevant section about your learning needs in the empty template on pages 148–158 if you are working on your own personal development plan, or to the practice or workplace personal and professional development plan on pages 174–181 if you are working on a practice or workplace team learning plan. Don't forget to keep the evidence of your learning in your personal portfolio.

References

1 Public Health Laboratory Service, Department of Health and Social Security and PS, Scottish ISD(D) 5 Collaborative Group (2000) *Trends in Sexually Transmitted Infections in the United Kingdom, 1990 to 1999*. Public Health Laboratory Service, London; *see also* http://www.phls.co.uk.

2 Department of Health (1992) *The Health of the Nation*. HMSO, London.

3 Adler MW (1988) *ABC of Sexually Transmitted Diseases*. BMJ Books, London.

4 http://www.agum.org.uk

5 Barton S (2000) *Clinical Evidence. Issue 5*. BMJ Books, London; *see also* http://www.clinicalevidence.org

6 Joint Formulary Committee (2001) *British National Formulary*. British Medical Association and Royal Pharmaceutical Society of Great Britain, London.

7 Lamagni TL, Hughes G, Rogers PA *et al.* (1999) New cases seen in genitourinary medicine clinics: England 1998. *Commun Dis Rep CDR Suppl.* **9**: S1–12.

8 Community Disease Surveillance Council (2000) AIDS and HIV in the United Kingdom: monthly report. *Commun Dis Rep CDR Weekly.* **10**: 37.

9 Greenhouse P (1994) A sexual health service under one roof: setting up sexual health services for women. *J Matern Child Health.* **19**: 228–33.

10 Chambers R (2000) *Involving Patients and the Public: how to do it better*. Radcliffe Medical Press, Oxford.

CHAPTER 8

Managing sexual dysfunction in primary care

Presentation

Sexual dysfunction is common in the general population.[1] The association of sexual difficulties with social functioning or psychological and physical ill health has been described,[2] but many of the studies of prevalence have been on selected clinic populations such as those with diabetes.[3] Some studies found very different prevalence rates for problems with sexual activity – for example, 20% in one from general medical practice[4] and 53% in another from a specialist arthritis department.[5]

Dunn's questionnaire survey of 4000 randomly selected patients in general practices found that the prevalence of one or more defined sexual dysfunctions was 44% in men and 36% in women.[6] Only 5% of those had received help from their general practitioner, but 42% would like help with their problem. The commonest choice of professional help was the family doctor, followed by the family planning clinic. Half of the women wanted help from a female professional, but only 27% of the men specified that they would prefer a male professional. This study indicated that sexual dysfunction was associated with self-reported physical problems in men, and with psychological and social problems in women. This implies that effective health promotion and sexual therapy could have a broad impact on health in the adult population, and that people felt that primary care was the setting where they wished to consult about their sexual dysfunction. Some consultations are more appropriate than others. For example, a consultation for acute lower abdominal pain in a woman who has had two children is not the best time to make a psychosexual exploration of her reply that she has not had sexual intercourse for several months.

Self-referral occurs either with an openly presented problem, or with a hidden problem (*see* below). The patient has chosen to consult a health professional rather than a relationship therapist, counsellor or religious adviser. Patients who consult doctors and nurses expect holistic care, including an examination of their mind, body and social circumstances.

Referral by the patient's partner

If the patient remarks that their sexual partner has told them to attend, it is important to establish whether they perceive there to be a problem, too. If the person attending does not feel that there is a problem, does the absent partner expect or hope that the doctor or nurse will tell the patient to change? You may need to see the partner instead, but it is important to be careful that you are not colluding with the patient in front of you into blaming the absent partner. You may end up with two people each blaming the other for the difficulty or problem.

The consultation

Unease about discussing the area of sexuality can discourage practitioners from even approaching the subject. The more often you signal to patients that you are prepared to talk about sex and that you are comfortable with the subject, the easier it will be for them to share their concerns. Problems may be either presented openly or hidden behind other opening gambits (*see* Table 8.1).

Patients are often unsure of the reception that they will receive from the health professional and may try out these strategies to establish whether it is acceptable to mention their problems.

Table 8.1 Presentation of sexual problems

Overt presentation	*Hidden presentation*
Lack of desire (libido)	The visiting card of another complaint
Lack of performance	The hand on the door on the way out
Lack of satisfaction	The oblique approach (dropping hints)
Occasionally too much desire or a perversion	Somatic complaints or surrogate markers such as recurrent discharge or pain

---

Box 8.1

Mrs N presented with complaints of various aches and pains. She had not attended a doctor for several years, and the doctor was puzzled about why she had come now with what appeared to be trivial problems. Having dealt with the presenting problems, the doctor asked if there was anything else, and was then asked a tentative question about symptoms of the menopause. It was not until the next appointment, when Mrs N returned to discuss the information she had been given about the menopause, that she revealed that she found sexual intercourse painful.

Similarly, patients who are unsure of their reception may postpone the presentation of the sexual problem until they are on the point of leaving, when they may blurt out a question about a sexual difficulty. At that stage a flight reaction is open for either the health professional or the patient. If the question is met by an annoyed or alarmed look from the doctor or nurse, the patient can say something like 'Oh, never mind', or 'I'll ask about that another time', and leave. The doctor or nurse can put up a defence – for example, by looking at the clock and remarking 'I can't deal with that today' – and see the patient leave with a sense of relief. A more welcoming response would be to deal with the question then and there by inviting the patient back to the chair to start again – if there is time to do so. If time is pressing, then an acknowledgement of the patient's difficulty, such as 'I can see this is important for you – it's difficult to ask about, isn't it?', and a firm arrangement to return to discuss it further, is more appropriate. Patients may present with complaints of abdominal or genital pain, or sometimes complaints in less closely related areas, hoping that an opportunity will arise to mention their sexual concerns. Sexual problems are more likely to be encountered when cervical cancer screening, contraceptive advice, mammography or testicular self-examination are being discussed. The prevention of transmission of common infections such as chlamydia, the prevention of pelvic inflammatory disease in young women, and the detection of subclinical sexually transmitted diseases in men are all conditions for which discussion of sexual matters is essential.

If you are to take a competent sexual history, you need to be careful not to assume that you know what the problem is. It is easy to jump to conclusions, to think that this patient is like the last one you saw, and that the solutions that you propose will be suitable.[7]

Box 8.2

Mrs B was referred to a menopause clinic for advice, as she complained that she had lost her libido since her periods stopped three years ago. Her GP had tried several different regimes of HRT with no benefit. The gynaecologist at the clinic had confidently told her that an implant of testosterone would do the trick, but now she was back with no improvement at all. Her GP asked the practice nurse if she would see her to 'support her through'. The practice nurse reported that she took a full history again, listening actively to the patient. She had asked what else had happened three years ago and heard a different story. Mrs B's father had died three years ago, and Mrs B and her husband had fallen out over the demands that had been made by her difficult, disabled and manipulative mother ever since. Her husband made acid remarks about having to get his own tea, while she got her mother's. She was helped to see how she could learn to manage her mother's demands and establish communication again with her husband – and her libido returned as she was able to see herself again as a person and a wife, and not just as a daughter or carer.

Most people will be able to tell you what the problem is and, by looking at it with you, discover what is the right thing for *them* to do to put it right.

By the end of the account by the patient you will usually know the following:

- when the problem started (i.e. whether the problem is primary or secondary)
- if anything happened at the time when it started (could this be causally related or is it a 'red herring'?)
- if it always happens or if it is associated with any particular circumstance or person (this may help with identifying difficult personal relationships or environments)
- why the person has presented now (is it due to pressure from a partner, a trigger from changed circumstances, etc.).

If you have not identified any of these factors, pay attention to the reasons why this is so. The patient may be putting up a defence because he or she does not want to tell you.

Box 8.3

Mr L was very vague in his account of his problems. He complained of loss of erection 'sometimes', but was curiously evasive about when this occurred. The doctor felt confused. Eventually she said to him that she was not clear exactly when he was having the difficulty, as he seemed to be saying he was not having a problem most of the time. After a short silence he sought reassurance that the consultation was confidential and that no one else would be told. The doctor explained that the information received would remain confidential unless someone else's life or health was clearly at risk. Mr L then explained that it only happened when he tried to use a condom on his 'nights out with the boys' when he ended up with a one-night stand. An attractive man, he had no difficulty in picking up a girl at nightclubs, but was afraid that his mates would find out that he was not the stud he appeared to be. He thought that the doctor would be critical of his behaviour – as indeed he was of himself when challenged, and feared that his wife would find out how he had been behaving.

A woman may not tell you that she had exciting orgasmic sex with a previous partner if she is afraid that her present partner will discover that she compares him unfavourably. You may not be told something significant that happened at the time when the problem started because it seems either too trivial or too terrible to mention.

Be an active thinking listener, not a passive receptacle for information. Pay attention to what is going on between you and the patient. Does it shed any light on how that patient relates to others outside the room?

The urgent appointment may mean that the complaint is urgent (e.g. premature ejaculation) or that the attention needed is urgent (e.g. the girlfriend is leaving if he doesn't get the difficulty sorted out). Sometimes it is a sign of ambivalence – the patient only wants to spare a short period of time, or knows that the health professional will only have a short amount of time, so there is plenty of opportunity for flight.

The 'non-urgent' appointment can also indicate ambivalence (e.g. 'I'm not sure that I want to look at this, so I will have an appointment in six weeks' time') or low self-esteem (e.g. 'I know you are too busy to pay attention to my silly needs').

The 'special' appointment is interesting and often irritating, when the health professional realises that the patient has successfully manipulated them into arranging to see them outside normal consulting hours or for much longer than usual. Even more irritating, but in need of understanding, is the specially arranged appointment that is not attended. Is this due to ambivalence, a sense of worthlessness, more manipulation, anger or just plain forgetfulness?

Examination

Patients often want a physical examination, and at the very least they should be offered one. If you find yourself avoiding a physical examination, this is a significant finding in its own right. What is it about a physical examination that is so difficult with *this* patient? Is it the patient's fear of what you might find – too terrible to be shown, so small that you might ridicule it (the vagina or the penis), too young (emotionally) to be examined, or a repeat of previous abuse? Consider offering the patient a chaperone to be present in the room. Although this may be difficult in practice, and may inhibit the patient from opening up about intimate matters during the examination, it is important that they feel that you are sensitive to their needs.

A physical examination that is accepted or welcomed by the patient can be very helpful. You may find a physical reason for the problem, or the absence of a finding (e.g. pain) can help the patient to face the possibility of a psychological cause. Occasionally a physical examination can help the patient to talk about things that they would otherwise have concealed – as if taking off the clothes also helps to remove other barriers. Be an *active* listener during the physical examination, and use the non-verbal clues just as much as in the history taking. Be purposeful and systematic in the examination, exactly as you would be for any other examination (*see* Boxes 8.4 and 8.5). Just because it is an examination for a sexual complaint does not mean that it is any less clinical or professional. Explain exactly what you are doing during the examination. The patient should be quite clear about the normality or otherwise of the examination as you proceed, and you should ensure that they understand why you are doing each part. Examining the prostate or inspecting the clitoris may be obvious steps to you, but can be misunderstood by a patient unless you communicate the reasons and the findings in the context of the problem.

Box 8.4 Male examination[8]

General inspection	• Non-verbal clues about depression, anxiety, hypomania, etc.
	• Distribution of facial and body hair or gynaecomastia for signs of androgen deficiency or other endocrine abnormality
	• Breathlessness due to respiratory disease when undressing or talking, which may limit the ability to be active during sexual activity
Cardiovascular	• Blood pressure, peripheral pulses, other signs of arteriosclerosis or raised lipid levels
Musculoskeletal	• Difficulty in getting undressed or on to the couch, indicating problems with flexibility during intercourse
Nervous system	• The history may indicate a problem with the lumbosacral innervation, so check for sensation in the perineal or lower limbs if indicated
Abdominal	• Evidence of abdominal surgery and the emotions expressed about the scars may be relevant
	• Palpable bladder may indicate a prostate problem
	• Hernias can cause pain or obstruction to intercourse
Genital	• Note and discuss with the patient the appearance of the genitals
	• The size of the flaccid penis is very variable (5–10 cm) and may seem smaller in obese men. Many men think that their penis is 'too small'
	• Assess any thickened plaques if Peyronie's disease is suggested by a history of a bend in the erect penis
	• Retract the foreskin, if present, and note any pain, scarring or restriction – tears of the frenulum are a common cause of painful sex in young men
	• Exclude any STI (e.g. warts)

	• The testes should feel smooth and symmetrical; small epididymal cysts are common and can be tender; a varicocoele or a hernia may also produce tenderness above the testes
Prostate	• Assess for irregularity, asymmetry or hardness (suggestive of a malignancy) or tenderness (suggestive of prostatitis)
Rectal	• For anal warts, haemorrhoids or a fissure

Box 8.5 Female examination[8]

General inspection	• Signs of mental distress or abnormality as for male examination
	• Development of secondary sexual characteristics
	• Exclude hirsutism or other signs of virilisation
	• Breathlessness due to respiratory disease when undressing or talking, which may limit the ability to be active during sexual activity
Cardiovascular	• Blood pressure, peripheral pulses, other signs of arteriosclerosis or raised lipid levels, although of uncertain aetiology in arousal disorders in women
Musculoskeletal	• Osteoarthritis of the hips with loss of external rotation or back pain is a common cause of difficulty in older women
Nervous system	• Loss of sensations or reflexes in the perineal area is rare, but may occur in multiple sclerosis or spinal nerve damage
Abdominal	• Evidence of abdominal surgery and the emotions expressed about the scars may be relevant
	• Irritable bowel syndrome with pain from pressure on the distended or tender gut is a common cause of dyspareunia
	• Extensive pelvic surgery may damage the pelvic nerves

Genital	• Note and discuss with the patient the appearance of the genitals • Assess for urinary stress incontinence if indicated by the history • A digital examination can confirm or exclude pain. A pain-free digital examination when the complaint is dyspareunia is particularly helpful • Assess for adequate oestrogenisation • Any signs of STI or of irritation or thrush. Take swabs if indicated; chlamydia in particular is indicated in complaints of dyspareunia • Gynaecological abnormalities (e.g. fibroids or ovarian cysts) may indicate a referral for further assessment

Investigations

Be guided by the history. You would not check the prolactin level or visual field in everyone, just because some people with pituitary disorders have sexual problems before other symptoms. Similarly, you would not consider performing a test of the testosterone level in a young man who has sudden-onset erectile dysfunction after his girlfriend has gone off with his best friend.

Box 8.6 Investigations[8]

1 *Testosterone level at 9 a.m.*: low levels in the morning usually suggest hypogonadism in men.
2 *Serum hormone binding globulin*: to calculate the free androgen index (if available).
3 *Luteinising hormone level*: low levels suggest a pituitary problem, and a raised level suggests testicular or ovarian failure.
4 *Prolactin level*: raised levels may be iatrogenic or indicate a pituitary problem. If levels are only mildly raised, it may not be significant, and the test should be repeated.

5   Other tests suggested by the history may include the following:
- follicle-stimulating hormone and luteinising hormone to establish whether a woman is menopausal (especially if the patient has had a hysterectomy or has amenorrhoea at under 50 years of age)
- thyroid hormone and thyroid-stimulating hormone levels
- liver function tests (if drug or alcohol abuse is suspected)
- biochemical screening or full blood count (e.g. in complaints of fatigue to exclude physical illness such as leukaemia or Addison's disease)
- prostate-specific antigen if prostatic disease is suspected.

Sometimes you need to perform blood tests so that the patient can start to move away from only considering physical causes. Be a 'whole-person health professional'. For example, it would be negligent not to check the blood sugar level in a 50-year-old man with gradual onset of erectile dysfunction, or to fail to perform a thyroid function test in someone who is complaining of a lack of libido, weight gain, thinning hair and dry skin.

Loss of desire

This is the commonest complaint in women, but it represents a whole spectrum of disorders, and often also occurs in men. The complaint may always have been present and so not really be a loss, but rather a lack of desire for sexual activity. It may represent inhibition – that is, repression of sexual thoughts due to feelings of being too young (whatever the chronological age), too pure (sex is dirty or unsuitable in some way) or forbidden (by upbringing or religious taboo). It may represent a lack of compatibility in the expectations of the couple – either real or due to beliefs in myths (see Box 8.7).

Box 8.7 Some of the myths about sex that people believe in (even when they say they don't!)

- Men are always ready for sex.
- Men do not show or talk about their emotions.
- A lover always knows how his or her partner feels without having to ask or be told.

- Men should always take the lead, initiate and orchestrate sexual activity.
- It is a man's job to satisfy the woman and bring her to orgasm.
- All physical contact between a couple leads to sexual activity.
- Sexual activity always involves penile penetration of the vagina leading to ejaculation.
- Sexual activity should be natural and spontaneous, and should never be planned or set up.
- Failure to achieve erection or orgasm is a disaster and means that the person concerned does not love/desire the partner.
- Everyone should be able to have successful sexual intercourse without practising or learning how to do it better.
- Both members of a couple will always feel ready to have sex at the same time.

The woman may believe in the myth of the 'ever-ready' man, or the man may feel let down by the lack of interest shown by his wife when she is absorbed and tired out by the demands of a new baby. The natural settling down into a less sexually active routine after the exciting first 6 to 12 months of a new relationship can be interpreted as a loss of interest in or by the partner.

Life events have a powerful effect on sexual functioning and sexual problems are more likely to occur at critical times such as the following:

- beginning sexual life
- getting married
- having a baby
- having adolescents at home
- children leaving home
- losses (e.g. of job, parents, health, youthfulness, opportunities, partners, etc.)
- moving into old age or what the person perceives to be old age
- reminders of old psychological damage, such as sexual or emotional abuse.

Some medical problems may make loss of desire more likely or be causative (see Box 8.8). Be cautious about laying the blame in this direction, as it may be a false clue or a source of false assumptions.

Many people who are seriously or chronically ill will not be interested in sexual activity – but for others it is an important and essential reaffirmation of their love for each other even when one of them is terminally ill.

Box 8.8 Medical factors to consider in loss of desire

Illnesses	Medications
Pain on intercourse, due to gynaecological, obstetric or urological disorders	Anti-androgens (e.g. cyproterone gonadotrophin-releasing-hormone analogues)
Alcohol or illegal drug misuse	Anti-oestrogens (e.g. tamoxifen), some contraceptives*
Stress or chronic anxiety	Cytotoxic drugs
Endocrine disorders (e.g. pituitary tumours, hypothyroidism, possibly diabetes)	Psychoactive drugs e.g. sedatives, narcotics, antidepressants, neuroleptics, stimulants)
Neurological disorders (e.g. hypothalamic disease, stroke)	
Depression or phobias	

* *Psychological reasons are more common than pharmacological ones with oral contraceptive use.*

Looking at the circumstances of the difficulty *for a particular couple or individual* helps them to make sense of the situation and what they might do to modify or remedy the underlying causes. Sometimes the cause may be loss of attraction for, or even dislike of, the partner. If the health professional dislikes the partner from the description given, perhaps the patient does too! Relationship therapy may be an option for motivated couples, or sometimes the patient just needs to come to terms with the realisation that the partnership has to end. More often it is a combination of several small adjustments in attitudes, thought patterns, assumptions or behaviour that can be made by an individual or a couple that helps the complainant to move towards a resolution or acceptance of the problem.

Lack of performance

Erectile dysfunction represents a large part of the work concerned with sexual dysfunction presented in primary care, and has more options for treatment. For these reasons it has a chapter to itself (*see* Chapter 9).

Lack of orgasm is commoner in women than in men. In men it tends to occur as retarded or lack of ejaculation, mostly in men who have difficulty in expressing their emotions, often due to fear of loss of control, or who are over-controlling themselves for some psychological gain. Other causes include antidepressant or antipsychotic drug treatment, or neurological damage.[9] Retrograde ejaculation may be misinterpreted as lack of ejaculation, and is most common after prostatectomy, although it may occur in otherwise healthy men.

Orgasmic dysfunction in women is often linked to myths about the responsibility of the male partner to be able to produce the orgasm 'for the woman'. Fears or inhibitions about masturbation may have prevented a woman from discovering how to produce an orgasm herself, or she may have been unable to transfer this experience to heterosexual activity. Exploration of her own erotic areas, self-stimulation and better communication between the partners during sexual arousal and intercourse can lead to a resolution if the psychological barriers protecting the patient from hidden fears are not too great.

Vaginismus

Vaginismus is the *symptom* of a disorder in which spasm of the vaginal muscles prevents the penis from entering the vagina, or only allows it to enter with pain or discomfort. Penetration may be impossible and the woman may be unable to:

- touch the vulva herself
- find any opening
- allow anyone else to touch it
- allow anything inside.

However, women with vaginismus can sometimes have a vaginal delivery after artificial insemination (i.e. a baby can come out, but the penis cannot enter).

Vaginismus may be primary (i.e. the woman has always been like this) or secondary. Secondary vaginismus will often have been caused by the experience of pain after infection, forced intercourse, a difficult delivery, imagined or real disfigurement after episiotomy, or any instrumentation in that area (whether vaginal, urethral or rectal).

Primary vaginismus is usually due to fear, and is similar to a panic disorder or phobia. This condition is not amenable to an operation under anaesthetic to 'open it up', however tempting it may be to think in these mechanistic terms. Many women with minor problems can be helped both by advice and by learning how to explore their own vagina to remove the fear of the unknown. Others have a more complex phobia and fantasies, the overcoming of which can take many months of gradual progress and constant testing of the fear or fantasy against reality. Remember that the fear and fantasy may prevent you from examining a vagina that is occasionally not normal and does have a physical barrier to overcome, but this will become apparent during the course of treatment.

Box 8.9

Both Mrs M and Mrs C had been attending the doctor for several months, gradually progressing from being unable to tolerate a finger on the vulva to being able to partially insert fingers and a plastic vaginal trainer into the vagina. Both women felt that there was something 'in the way' higher up. They both happened to attend the doctor in the same week and were able for the first time to allow examination. Mrs M's vagina was normal and the cervix was clearly visualised with a speculum after digital examination. Mrs C's vagina felt different, and examination with a speculum showed a partial septum and a tiny second cervix. She had a bifid uterus, but the doctor recalled another patient with a similar abnormality whom she had seen for an intrauterine device fitting after a normal vaginal delivery – no vaginal spasm there!

Vulval pain

Superficial vulval pain is common and has a multiplicity of possible underlying factors, including the following:

- vulvitis or vulvovaginitis from infection
- vulval vestibulitis – an inflammation around the vestibular area with severe pain to the touch[10]

- vulvodynia – a condition of persisting pain of unknown aetiology possibly related to post-viral infection sensitivity or psychological fears, which may overlap with vestibulitis
- genital herpes
- urethritis
- atrophic vulvitis
- inadequate lubrication
- irritants such as spermicides, detergents, scents, dyes or sweat.

Although the majority of women have short-lived symptoms which can be relieved by treatment of the underlying cause, a few continue to suffer considerable distress. Some cases resolve (after exclusion of infection) with graduated reducing doses of topical steroids. For others the condition may be part of a psychological defence, and a few cases remain 'medically unexplained' even after specialist referral and investigation.

Referral

Ideally, referral onward occurs when the patient and the health professional agree to seek a specialist opinion or to obtain more specialist investigations or treatment.

Patients may not wish to discuss their private sexual life with someone they see for other physical complaints, and ask for a referral for this reason. However, it is still important to establish what the problem is and who is the most relevant professional to help them.

Health professionals may have their own fears or difficulties with confusion of roles, especially if they know the patient socially. It can be a sensible conclusion to refer if it would cause awkwardness to do otherwise, but it is worth trying to understand your own motives. If you could cope with knowing other types of secrets about a patient, but not the sexual ones, the problem may be yours and not the patient's.

You can only refer the patient for expert help if you know who the experts are. Meeting and talking with the staff from the range of facilities in your area is the best way of being able to discuss with patients who would be the best choice for their particular problem. You cannot meet them all, but you should at least know what type of treatment is on offer.

Reflection exercises

Exercise 24

The doctors and nurses might discuss who they feel should be identifying and offering help to patients with sexual problems (often each thinks it is the other's job). If they are involved in providing other services, such as contraception, investigation of STIs, screening for chlamydia and other activities related to sexual health, they may feel that greater expertise is needed. Find out what facilities are available for extra training and education in your area from university departments or from national organisations such as the British Association of Sexual and Relationship Therapy or the Institute of Psychosexual Medicine (*see* list of useful addresses on page 133).

Exercise 25

Do you know what referral facilities are available for sexual or relationship problems in your area? If your practice team or clinic does not have a suitable resource list, perhaps the secretary, receptionist or another member of staff could investigate and draw one up. You might involve all members of the wider team in the investigation in order to find as many different sources of help as possible – from voluntary and religious groups as well as health service provision. You might investigate how other practices or clinics have made provision for a Relate therapist to work at their premises, and find out what services have been purchased from secondary care.

> Now that you have completed these interactive reflection exercises, transfer the information to the relevant section about your learning needs in the empty template on pages 148–158 if you are working on your own personal development plan, or to the practice or workplace personal and professional development plan on pages 174–181 if you are working on a practice or workplace team learning plan. Don't forget to keep the evidence of your learning in your personal portfolio.

Useful addresses

British Association of Sexual and Relationship Therapy, PO Box 13686, London SW20 9ZH. Website: www.basrt.org.uk

Institute of Psychosexual Medicine, 12 Chandos Street, Cavendish Square, London W1D 9DR. Website: www.ipm.org.uk

References

1 Lewin J and King M (1997) Sexual medicine: towards an integrated discipline. *BMJ.* **314**: 1432.

2 Ussher JM and Baker CD (eds) (1993) *Psychological Perspectives on Sexual Problems.* Routledge, London.

3 Hackett GI (1995) Impotence: the most neglected complication of diabetes. *Diabetes Res.* **28**: 75–83.

4 Ende J, Rockwell S and Glasgow M (1984) The sexual history in general medical practice. *Arch Intern Med.* **144**: 558–61.

5 Blake DJ, Weaver W, Maisiak R *et al.* (1990) A curriculum in clinical sexuality for arthritis care professionals. *Acad Psychosom Med.* **2**: 189–91.

6 Dunn KM, Croft PR and Hackett GT (1999) Association of sexual problems with social, psychological and physical problems in men and women: a cross-sectional population study. *J Epidemiol Commun Health.* **53**: 144–8.

7 Skrine R and Montford H (eds) (2001) *Psychosexual Medicine: an introduction.* Edward Arnold, London.

8 Tomlinson J (ed.) (1999) *ABC of Sexual Health.* BMJ Books, London.

9 Bancroft J (1989) *Human Sexuality and its Problems.* Churchill Livingstone, Edinburgh.

10 Maurice WL (1999) *Sexual Medicine in Primary Care.* Mosby Inc., St Louis, MO.

CHAPTER 9

Erectile dysfunction (impotence)

What is erectile dysfunction?

Erectile dysfunction (ED) is the inability to produce and maintain an erection that is sufficient for penetrative sexual intercourse. Erection occurs when the penile smooth muscle is relaxed by stimulation of the parasympathetic nervous system. Central sensory stimulation and/or penile stimulation initiates the erection. Biochemically the relaxation is mediated by activating the biochemical pathways to increase the blood flow through the penile arteries. The rise in intracavernous pressure flattens and obstructs the venous outflow, thereby producing rigidity.

All men experience a failure of erection at some time, but continuing difficulty is rare in men under 40 years of age. The incidence increases rapidly thereafter, with about 65% of men over 70 years of age having difficulty. The increase is mainly due to reductions in vascular flow, but occurs about 10 years earlier in men with diabetes, possibly because of the additional contribution of parasympathetic nerve disturbances. With increasing age, most men find that they require more stimulation to produce an erection, it may be less firm than it used to be, and they lose the erection more easily if they are distracted.

Causes

Cardiovascular disease and diabetes are probably the commonest physical causes of erectile dysfunction (*see* Table 9.1), but taking medication (more likely with increasing age), may also affect function (*see* Table 9.2).

Table 9.1 Causes of erectile dysfunction (except medication)

Psychological	Circulatory	Neurological	Endocrine
Anxiety	Arteriosclerosis	Spinal or pelvic	Androgen
Depression	Hyperlipidaemia	trauma	deficiency
Loss	Smoking	Radical pelvic	Hyperprolactinaemia
Relationship	Diabetes	surgery	Thyroid disorders
problems	Hypertension	Multiple	
		sclerosis	
		Diabetes	
		Alcohol	
		Nerve root	
		compression	

Remember that it is a whole person who has the problem. Even if the problem started as a physically related one, the man (and his partner) will have feelings about it which contribute to the difficulty.

Table 9.2 Drugs associated with erectile dysfunction

Antihypertensives	Antidepressants	Tranquillisers	Other medication	Recreational
Thiazides	Tricyclics	Phenothiazines	Anti-androgens	Heroin
Beta-blockers	Monoamine	Thioxanthenes	Cimetidine	Drugs
Central alpha-	oxidase	Butyrophenones	Clofibrate	substituting
blockers	inhibitors	Diazepam	Digoxin	for orgasmic
Others*	Fluoxetine		Indomethacin	activity
				Anabolic
				steroids
				Alcohol
				Tobacco

* All antihypertensive drugs may cause impotence by lowering the pressure in arteriosclerotic vessels, but some have a greater effect than would be expected from this alone.

The consultation

The history

First you need to establish exactly what the problem is. Many men describe their sexual problem as 'impotence' when it is in fact premature ejaculation or loss of libido. Just as with any condition, find out the following information:

- when it started – a gradual onset suggests a mainly physical cause, whereas a sudden onset usually has a psychological cause
- whether anything else happened at about the same time – e.g. loss of a job, loss of a relationship or relative, a new baby, retirement, an episode of ill health, etc.
- why he is coming to see you about it at this time – has it just started?; has the partner threatened to leave?; did he read or hear about treatment that he did not think was available before, etc.?
- whether it only happens at certain times – e.g. with one partner but not with another, with a partner but not with masturbation, at home but not on holiday, etc.
- what his general health is like and whether any symptoms suggest particular causes (*see* Table 9.1) or require investigation
- whether he is taking any drugs that you do not know about – e.g. alcohol, anabolic steroids.

Most of the time, people will provide you with all of this information without any prompting. If you notice that you have not been told something, you should consider whether the information has been concealed out of fear, for example, that you might disapprove, or think them foolish or too old.

The examination

Patients often comment on how enormously helpful a physical examination is for them. It makes them feel that you are taking the situation seriously and that you are looking at them as an individual and as a whole person. It is rare to find any physical abnormality (e.g. hypogonadism, lichen sclerosis of the foreskin, scleroderma or a massive hernia) getting in the way – but it does happen. More often the examination gives you a chance to observe how the man feels about his genitals. For example, he may remark how small they are, or gesture angrily at his penis because it refuses to work, or he may just appear sad or anxious as he looks at them. Reflecting back the emotional content can give you a greater understanding of the situation.

Box 9.1

A 49-year-old man said that he had had poor erections since his hernia repair and thought perhaps 'they had caught a nerve'. When the female doctor suggested an examination, he looked very anxious. During the examination he looked away at the wall, detaching himself. When the doctor made an observation about this, he flushed and was able to tell her that he had had the beginnings of an erection when his stitches were removed. The nurse had been quite sharp with him and told him to cover himself up. The doctor remarked that the nurse 'had put him down' and the patient looked thoughtful. He returned for the results of his (normal) blood sugar test and told the doctor that he had had no further trouble. He said that being examined and told he was all right must have made the difference.

The consultation also gives you an opportunity to check the blood pressure in someone who may not normally attend for routine checks. Any other examination (cardiovascular, neurological, prostate, etc.) will be dictated by the history.

Investigations

Just as in any other condition, investigations should be guided by the history. The sudden onset of impotence in a healthy young man whose partner has been unfaithful does not require investigations. A blood sugar test is essential for a man aged 44 years with a gradual onset of erectile difficulties and vague ill health. If abnormal results are found, they are not necessarily aetiological and may only be part of the problem. A man with a normal testosterone level feels just as keenly that he is 'less of a man' as another with a low result.

Box 9.2

Mr J had a prostatectomy. At his follow-up appointment, the urologist enquired about any sexual difficulties. He admitted to difficulty with erections, and a battery of tests was performed. A low testosterone level was found and he was started on replacement therapy. When he saw his GP he asked if he could stop the treatment. On enquiring a little further, the GP discovered that Mr J had always had difficulty with erections, and he and his wife of 30 years' standing had 'found ways round it', as Mr J put it. They did not want to change their habits now, and his erection was no better since his testosterone levels had been 'normalised'. He had been reading up on the treatment and was concerned about the risk of prostate cancer or a return of his enlarged prostate. After discussion, he decided to have a bone scan for osteoporosis, and if this was normal he would stop the testosterone.

Screening tests

Some authorities would propose that a battery of tests should always be performed, while others suggest that only those indicated by the history should be carried out. If practitioners initiate *screening* procedures, they should have conclusive evidence that screening can alter the natural history of that disease in a significant proportion of those screened[1] (*see* Chapter 6 on screening). The *ABC of Sexual Health* suggests that the basic investigations for most patients with an otherwise normal history will only involve checking the blood pressure and the blood sugar level.[2] Guidelines for the management of erectile dysfunction appear in the *Guidelines* publication or website of summary of guidelines for primary care.[3]

Occasionally, disorders of *desire* (loss of libido) can be linked with hormonal problems or be secondary to physical illness. It is worth screening for these because they are treatable and sometimes serious, difficult to differentiate on the basis of history alone, easy to detect with a blood test, and not costly compared with not testing. However, patients with erectile dysfunction often expect that the cause of their problem will be hormonal, and they cannot move on to discussing other factors until you have dealt with this possibility. A random testosterone test is normal in a high proportion of patients. If a low result is obtained (laboratory normal ranges vary) then further tests are indicated (*see* Box 8.6).

If it is thought that vascular function may be compromised, arrange additional investigations such as arteriography or Doppler ultrasound, or observe the response to injected drugs.

Opinions vary as to whether measuring nocturnal tumescence is reliable or useful. A portable monitor such as a Rigiscan is available for use by patients at home, but it is difficult to establish how reliable the results are, or even what part nocturnal tumescence plays in the evaluation of erectile dysfunction. It is not much comfort to a patient to know that nocturnal tumescence occurs if there is no erection while he is awake!

Any neurological symptoms should be confirmed by physical examination if possible.

Specialist referral may be required if the condition has not already been evaluated.

Treatment

Discuss the options for treatment (*see* Box 9.3). Establish that the man is fit enough to undertake sexual intercourse – if he can climb two flights of stairs, he is fit enough. If he is not fit enough to take an active role, you need to discuss alternatives to penetrative sexual intercourse, or taking a more passive role than he has done in the past. Discuss what he has talked to his partner about, and their expectations of treatment. A surprising number of men will not have discussed the issue with their partner at all. Some patients do not want any medical involvement, while others would prefer just to have treatment and no discussion of their feelings. Some reject an 'artificial' erection produced by treatment, and others just want to be able to say to their partner that they 'have done everything', while preferring to avoid sexual activity. Discuss how often they would like to use the treatment (e.g. the recommendations for alprostadil pellets are not more than twice in 24 hours and not more than seven times in 7 days). There will be constraints on how often the patient can have a prescription, either as a result of your own consideration of the drugs budget, or as a result of an agreement with your primary care organisation or pharmacist.

Box 9.3 Treatment options for erectile dysfunction

	Advantages	Disadvantages
Oral sildenafil Start with 50 mg; reduce to 25 mg if headache severe; increase to 100 mg if ineffective at lower dose	• Successful in 50–80% of cases • Non-invasive and simple to take • Few contra-indications • Few and usually tolerable side-effects (headache, dizziness, indigestion, blue-tinged vision)	• Depends on erotic stimulation to work – helps to produce the erection rather than acting as an instigator • Contraindicated for those taking nitrates or with a history of recent stroke or myocardial infarction, severe hepatic impairment, hypotension or hereditary retinal disorders • Slower action than alprostadil
Sublingual apomorphine Start with 2 mg, and increase to no more than 3 mg (other oral treatments will be available soon)	• Rapid onset, within about 20 minutes • Unaffected by food • No interactions with nitrates • Few side-effects (nausea, headaches, dizziness)	• Cannot be taken with other centrally acting dopamine agonists or antagonists • Contraindicated in patients with severe angina, recent myocardial infarction, severe heart failure or hypotension
Intracavernosal injections of alprostadil Adjust dose according to effectiveness, starting with 2.5 micrograms or 1.25 micrograms in cases of neurogenic impotence (other injections are still on trial at present)	• More effective than sildenafil • Few contra-indications • Rapid action • Produces a firm and sustained erection	• Penile pain is frequent (but usually mild) • Penile fibrosis may occur • Small risk of priapism (erection lasting longer than 4 hours and requiring surgical decompression) • Invasive; patients need to be taught precisely how to use it
Transurethral alprostadil Start with 250 micrograms and adjust to effective dose	• No needles • Less priapism than with injection • Few contra-indications	• Less effective than the injection • Penile discomfort and burning, sometimes also vaginal discomfort and burning • Slower-acting than injection • Requires dexterity and good eyesight to insert pellet into urethra after micturition

Vacuum devices	• No medication • Patient does not need to return to health professional • Can be continued long term by successful users	• Requires even more planning than other methods • Awkward and bulky to use • Erection can be uncomfortable, cold and appears blue • Erect penis pivots at the base, requiring care • Patient must remember to remove the constricting ring after intercourse • Contraindicated in bleeding disorders
Psychosexual therapy	• No physical invasion or medication • Can help to remove blocks to sexual activity • Can involve the partner, improving communication, sexual function and satisfaction	• People with skills in psychosexual therapy are only available in some areas • Patient may be reluctant to look at emotional component of problem • Can be time-consuming if problems are complex
Penile prosthesis	• Long-term result • Always available • Useful in cases of penile fibrosis • Cost of replacement is covered by guarantee	• Spontaneous erection can never return • Invasive operation with risk of infection and pain, and rarely erosion, migration of the prosthesis and penile necrosis • May show under clothing, as semirigid and malleable prostheses protrude • Mechanical problems (uncommon, but about 5% of cases)

In all but the last treatment option (penile prosthesis), spontaneous erections may return after initial treatment, especially in younger men with no cardiovascular or diabetic morbidity. Relieving the 'fear of failure' often leads to resolution of the problem and attention to the other underlying causes.

Advise the patient about avoidance of excess alcohol and quitting smoking, if applicable. Good diabetic control is sensible, and changing from one antihypertensive agent to another may occasionally be useful. Counselling and discussion help to make the man feel less abnormal, and may help to pinpoint any difficulties in the relationship that are contributing to the problem. Men with depression or other psychiatric disturbances need specific treatment, possibly with referral to secondary care. Reasons for referral are listed in Table 9.3.

Table 9.3 Patients who require referral from primary care

Problem	Facility
Hypogonadism or hyperprolactinaemia Poorly controlled diabetes	Endocrinologist
Neurological abnormalities or history suggestive of multiple sclerosis	Neurologist
Psychiatric illness (e.g. severe or continuing depression)	Psychiatrist
Relationship problems	Relate or other relationship counselling
Patient unwilling or unable to use physical therapies	Psychosexual counsellor
Patient request to examine emotional issues	Psychosexual counsellor
Patient requiring instruction in injection technique not available in primary care	Specialist provision, usually in urology, GUM or psychosexual departments
Failure of physical therapy, with request for prosthesis, or if penile fibrosis is present	Urologist

Most patients with erectile dysfunction can be successfully managed in primary care. Information on treatments and other useful advice can be obtained from the Impotence Association.[4]

The main management problem at present is the lack of availability of treatment on the NHS. At the time of writing, NHS prescriptions for erectile dysfunction treatments are restricted to men who:

- have diabetes, multiple sclerosis, Parkinson's disease, poliomyelitis, prostate cancer, severe pelvic injury, single-gene neurological disease, spina bifida or spinal cord injury
- are having renal dialysis
- have had radical pelvic surgery, prostatecomy or kidney transplant
- were receiving treatment at NHS expense on 14 September 1998.

In addition, specialist services commissioned by health authorities and primary care organisations, and operating under local agreements, may prescribe for men suffering 'severe distress' using hospital prescription forms.

Severe distress is defined as follows:

- significant disruption to normal social and occupational activities
- a marked effect on mood, behaviour, and social and environmental awareness
- a marked effect on interpersonal relationships.

Men who do not fall into the above categories have to pay for their treatment, with a private prescription being issued for the desired medication. Review of the regulations by the NHS is expected.

Reflection exercises

Exercise 26

Do you have suitable patient information leaflets that are easily accessible to patients who might be embarrassed to pick them up in public? Check that the information in the leaflets is up to date. They may still say things like 'no oral treatments for erectile dysfunction are available' when your patients know that this is not true (they have all heard of Viagra – sildenafil). Do you know who is responsible for the patient information leaflets and how often they are checked for accuracy? You may need to make some changes to ensure that supplies are accurate, accessible and replenished (see the exercises in Chapter 7 for suggestions as to how you might manage your patient information leaflets).

Exercise 27

You might arrange for a meeting at which a video of injection techniques is demonstrated by the local expert or specialist nurse, and to become more familiar with the instructions for other treatments. The practice team could discuss together how you manage requests for help from patients with erectile dysfunction, and whether the present arrangements are providing adequate access to treatment and equity between groups of patients. Define what improvements your practice team can make and what feedback you should give to your primary care organisation.

Exercise 28

You could be responsible for ensuring that others in the practice team are following accepted best practice for managing erectile dysfunction. The Impotence Association[4] produces a flow chart that is useful to work through when a patient presents with erectile dysfunction, or you could modify the guidelines to produce your own flow chart to meet your local requirements.

Exercise 29

Is everyone clear about the rationing of treatments for erectile dysfunction? You might wish to have a supply of leaflets explaining the current restrictions to give to patients. One such leaflet is available from the drug company that supplies sildenafil (Viagra), or you could write your own.

> Now that you have completed these interactive reflection exercises, transfer the information to the relevant section about your learning needs in the empty template on pages 148–158 if you are working on your own personal development plan, or to the practice or workplace personal and professional development plan on pages 174–181 if you are working on a practice or workplace team learning plan. Don't forget to keep the evidence of your learning in your personal portfolio.

References

1 Cochrane AL and Holland WW (1971) Validation of screening procedures. *Br Med Bull.* **27**: 3–8.
2 Tomlinson J (ed.) (1999) *ABC of Sexual Health.* BMJ Books, London.
3 Foord-Kelcey G (ed.) (2001) *Guidelines. Volume 13.* Medendium Group Publishing Ltd, Berkhamsted. Website: www.eguidelines.co.uk.
4 The Impotence Association, PO Box 10296, London SW17 9WH.

CHAPTER 10

Draw up and apply your personal development plan

Although you will probably want to focus on the clinical management of an aspect of sexual health, you may be interested in making the improvement of your prevention or management of any area of sexual health a focus of your personal development plan (PDP). A PDP on the prevention or management of an aspect of sexual health could supplement a practice personal and professional development plan on the same or other areas of sexual health (*see* Chapter 11). Therefore we have included a worked example of a personal development plan focused on the provision and management of contraceptive care as part of sexual health, on pages 159–171.

The example given is very comprehensive, and you may not want to include so much detail in your own personal development plan. You might include different topics and educational activities, because your needs and circumstances are different to those of the example practitioner here. You might want to spend 50% of your available time on this topic and the rest on other priority subjects such as those in National Service Frameworks, or topics from your local or district Health Improvement Programme.

You need to involve your colleagues and workplace team in anything that you propose including in your own personal development plan. Some suggestions are included in the example. You should also discuss it with your education and clinical governance leads in your own workplace, who will be able to help you focus on achievable aims and objectives, and also point out any gaps that you might not have thought about. Your personal development plan needs to feed into the practice or workplace development plans as well – so consult as widely as possible before you start. Keep it simple, so that after one year you will be able to measure some progress. Then you can build on that, or change focus for a while, in subsequent years.

Transfer the information about your learning needs from any of the reflection exercises at the end of the chapters that are relevant to you and that you have completed to the empty template of the personal development plan that follows on pages 148–158. The reflection exercises that you choose to select will depend on the focus of your PDP – as in the worked example here – or on other facets of sexual health matters.

The conclusions that you have reached at the end of each exercise will feature in the action plan of your personal development plan. Some more ideas about the preliminary information you should be gathering for your personal development plan are given in the boxes of the template.

Template for your personal development plan

Photocopy the following pages and complete one chart per topic.

What topic have you chosen?

Who chose it?

Justify why this topic is a priority:

(i)   *A personal or professional priority?*

(ii) *A practice priority?*

(iii) *A district priority?*

(iv) *A national priority?*

Who will be included in your personal development plan?
(Anyone other than you? Employed staff, attached staff, others from outside the practice, patients?)

Who will collect the baseline information and how?

How will you identify your learning needs?
(How will you obtain this information and who will do it? Self-completion check-lists, discussion, appraisal, audit, patient feedback?)

What are the learning needs of the practice and how do they match your needs?

Is there any patient or public input to your personal development plan?

What are the aims of your personal development plan arising from the preliminary data-gathering exercise?

How might you integrate the 14 components of clinical govern-ance into your personal development plan focusing on the topic of . . . . ?

Establishing a learning culture:

Managing resources and services:

Establishing a research and development culture:

Reliable and accurate data:

Evidence-based practice and policy:

Confidentiality:

Health gain:

Coherent team:

Audit and evaluation:

Meaningful involvement of patients and the public:

Health promotion:

Risk management:

Accountability and performance:

Core requirements:

Action learning plan (include timetabled action and expected outcomes)

How does your personal development plan tie in with your other strategic plans?
(For example, the practice's business or development plan, the local Health Improvement Programme or the Primary Care Investment Plan)

What additional resources will you require to execute your plan and from where do you hope to obtain them?
(Will you have to pay any course fees? Will you be able to organise any protected time for learning in working hours?)

How will you evaluate your personal development plan?

How will you know when you have achieved your objectives?
(How will you measure success?)

How will you disseminate the learning from your plan to the rest of the practice team and patients? How will you sustain your new-found knowledge or skills?

How will you handle new learning requirements as they crop up?

Check whether the topic you have chosen is a priority and the way in which you plan to learn about it is appropriate.

Photocopy this proforma for future use.

Your topic:

How have you identified your learning need(s)?

(*a*) PCO requirement ☐

(*b*) Practice business plan ☐

(*c*) Legal mandatory requirement ☐

(*d*) Job requirement ☐

(*e*) Appraisal need ☐

(*f*) New to post ☐

(*g*) Individual decision ☐

(*h*) Patient feedback ☐

(*i*) Other ☐

Have you discussed or planned your learning needs with anyone else?

Yes ☐   No ☐   If so, who?

What are your learning need(s) and/or objective(s) in terms of the following?

Knowledge. What new information do you hope to gain to help you to do this?

Skills. What should you be able to do differently as a result of undertaking this learning in your development plan?

Behaviour/professional practice. How will this impact on the way in which you then do things?

Details and date of desired development activity:

Details of any previous training and/or experience that you have in this area/dates:

What is your current performance in this area compared with the requirements of your job?

Need significant ☐   Need some development ☐
development in this area   in this area

Satisfactory in this area ☐   Do well in this area ☐

What is the level of job relevance that this area has to your role and responsibilities?

Has no relevance to job ☐   Has some relevance ☐

Relevant to job ☐   Very relevant ☐

Essential to job ☐

Describe how the proposed education/training is relevant to your job:

Do you need additional support in identifying a suitable development activity?

Yes ☐   No ☐

If Yes, what do you need?

Describe the differences or improvements for you, your practice, PCO and/or NHS trust as a result of undertaking this activity:

Assess the priority of your proposed educational/training activity:

Urgent ☐   High ☐   Medium ☐   Low ☐

Describe how the proposed activity will meet your learning needs rather than any other type of course or training on the topic:

If you had a free choice, would you want to learn this?   Yes/No

If **No**, why not? (please circle all that apply)

Waste of time
I have already done it
It is not relevant to my work or career goals
Other

If **Yes**, what reasons that are most important to you? (put them in rank order)

To improve my performance
To increase my knowledge
To get promotion
I am just interested in it
To be better than my colleagues
To do a more interesting job
To enable me to be more confident
Because it will help me
Other

Record of your learning activities

Write in the topic, date, time spent and type of learning

	Activity 1	Activity 2	Activity 3	Activity 4
In-house formal learning				
External courses				
Informal and personal				
Qualifications and/or experience gained				

Worked example

Personal development plan focusing on the provision and management of contraceptive care

Who chose the topic?

It might be your own choice or that of someone in the practice or PCO team who thinks that you should have additional skills in the provision and management of contraceptive care.

Why is the topic a priority?

(i) *A personal or professional priority?* You may have chosen the provision and management of contraceptive care, seeing a need for it yourself or as an inevitable development in your work. You may have agreed as part of your work development, or as a requirement of a change in work duties or responsibilities. You may have volunteered after development in the provision and management of contraceptive care was identified as a practice or PCO need.

(ii) *A practice priority?* The practice may have a need for an in-house expert to provide best practice and reduce costs. Perhaps the practice has identified that fees for contraceptive care are lower than average, or that local provision has been inadequate. You may have received a complaint, or a patient of yours may have been the subject of a critical incident analysis. Patient need or a different skill mix in the practice may have increased the need for expertise in the provision and management of contraceptive care.

(iii) *A district priority?* The PCO may need a local expert to provide guidelines and services, or they may have identified a need to reconsider how services are provided. They may be concerned about high referral rates to secondary care, or high termination or teenage pregnancy rates in the area.

(iv) *A national priority?* The reduction of unwanted conceptions, especially in younger teenagers, and the prevention of sexually transmitted illness represent an important national priority.

Who will be included in your personal development plan?

You might like to find others who want to increase their skills. Working together, or having a cascade of learning from each other, makes learning more cost-effective and you can set consistent standards of care. Learning skills and then passing them on makes for more effective learning for you, too.

Everyone needs to have the opportunity to increase their skills. Reception staff, the practice manager, secretaries, *all* of the health professionals and anyone who uses your premises might benefit from learning about the provision and management of contraceptive care. Disseminating basic information may reduce the workload of health professionals. Remember confidentiality and security issues.

You may want to consider training as a PCO activity to ensure consistency, exchange skills and reduce costs. Bringing in outside experts then becomes more cost-effective and can be tailormade for the particular needs of the learning group.

Who will collect the baseline information and how?

Ask the practice manager or secretary, or the clinical tutor at the PCO, the local contraceptive and sexual health community services, the gynaecology or genitourinary departments, or the Faculty of Family Planning and Reproductive Health Care of the Royal College of Obstetricians and Gynaecologists,[1] etc., for details of the training available. If you are already connected to the Internet, you can search for other more distant information yourself. Ask the facilities that you use for referral for feedback on your referrals (e.g. how appropriate they are, how you might modify your management before referral, etc.).

You need to know what is being done at present, so set up an audit of your present management. Find out the number of patients who are receiving contraceptive services in your practice, and in other practices in your PCO, and compare this with national standards. Establish what provision is already available for the various methods of contraception and the numbers of people using the services at present.

Find out what is in the pipeline for the immediate and long-term future development of the provision and management of contraceptive care in your area.

How will you identify your learning needs?

Among other methods, you might want to conduct a strengths, weaknesses, opportunities and threats (SWOT) analysis for yourself and with your practice team.

Strengths: enthusiasm; an interest in contraceptive care; willingness to go on learning; communication skills and inter-professional relationships to enable inter-disciplinary working; organisational, teaching and research skills to provide a resource for the management of contraceptive services; a practice with sufficient spare capacity for quality improvements and to provide a resource for the PCO.

Opportunities: a contact in contraceptive and sexual health services for the locality; an individual with skills in the provision and management of contraceptive care, who is enthusiastic about passing on his or her newly acquired knowledge; expertise in evaluating interventions is available on which you can build to improve professional proficiency; you have decided to develop expertise in provision of best contraceptive care.

Weaknesses and threats: deficiencies in equipment, time for carrying out services, and the availability of training; too many other guidelines and increasing numbers of National Service Framework requirements for the practice team to meet; other commitments, antagonism or lack of support from others, both inside the practice team, from other practices and outside the practice from secondary and community services.

You might include a survey of the expertise available in your PCO and elsewhere, and list the present competencies of other staff. What skills and services are accessible inside and outside your own workplace?

What are the learning needs of the practice and how do they match your needs?

The prioritising exercise should already have given you some information. Consider inviting people to express their concerns and opinions at a practice team meeting, or ask another member of staff to organise it. The practice manager could ask the practice team to complete a checklist of their own needs and wishes for the provision and management of contraceptive care, and what they would like from others. The clinical governance lead or development officer of the PCO could do the same for the district.

One staff member might wish to specialise and become an expert in the provision and management of contraceptive care. Does this fit with the requirements of the practice (or PCO)? Or would it be more cost-effective to use that expertise from another practice or from the existing community services?

A GP might wish to become an intermediate care provider for the PCO, or work in a community clinic or as a clinical assistant in secondary care. What implications does this have for the practice in terms of cover for clinical sessions?

A practice nurse might wish to gain expertise in and take over much of the contraceptive care for patients using hormonal methods of contraception and emergency contraception. What implications does this have for her or his other workload?

You might find that your local community clinic wishes to take over more of the management of sexual health matters and provide a resource for long-term methods of contraception and for medical gynaecology. Does this have implications for your budget and waiting-list for other conditions?

You might wish to employ a doctor or nurse with special expertise to supplement what is available within the practice, or to provide space for one to work independently at your practice. What does this mean for your patients? Can you recommend patients to attend? Who will pay for the service? Will it make a difference to the income from contraceptive fees? Will it be independent or managed by the practice? Will you need to make alterations to the layout of your premises, or to the equipment used? How will this be financed? Do you know what their qualifications mean and what level of service they might be expected to provide?

You might like the PCO to purchase, or arrange to use independently, services at a local clinic for the provision of particular methods of contraception, such as intrauterine devices or implants, or for the provision of termination of pregnancies or vasectomy and female sterilisation.

You may want to provide contraceptive services to all comers. This requires negotiation with other practices to make sure that they do not feel that you are 'poaching' their patients or taking their contraceptive fees.

Is there any patient or public input to your personal development plan?

You may well have some local experts who could help the practice. Think about how you would go about recruiting them and the implications for confidentiality.

Find out what patients think would be useful. Ask for feedback, organise a focus group or set up a representative local group.

You could set up evening or Saturday morning sessions or visit schools, youth clubs, working men's clubs or women's groups to publicise what is and will be available, and to obtain feedback on the current provision. Think about inviting a well-known local figure to one or two of the sessions to increase the impact and gain some free publicity (let the local newspaper or television/radio station know about your plans).

Arrange for computer terminals or poster displays that give access to other sources of advice provided by other agencies (e.g. libraries, Citizens' Advice Bureau, the Council).

What mechanism(s) will you use to find out the answers in a meaningful way, and not just from those who are most opinionated or compliant? You may need to think deeply about the reliability of any method, and how representative individual patients are of your practice population as a whole.

What are the aims of your personal development plan arising from the preliminary data-gathering exercise?

To learn how to:

- provide good primary care services for young people[2,3]
- ensure confidentiality[4]
- take an adequate sexual history[5,6]
- provide hormonal contraception in line with current best practice[7-9]
- increase the knowledge about availability of services among potential users
- be better informed about long-acting methods of contraception[10,11]
- increase your range of skills with regard to providing some long-term methods of contraception
- set up forms for automating the recording of clinical encounters, management and activity reports, annual report information, etc.
- identify the risk factors for common sexually transmitted infections and ways to minimise them
- identify best practice for investigation and treatment of vaginal discharge and other medical gynaecological conditions
- increase your skills in identifying psychosexual problems in contraceptive care[12]
- provide good patient leaflets and information
- set up ways of keeping yourself and other staff up to date with current thinking and best practice.

How might you integrate the 14 components of clinical governance into your personal development plan focusing on the topic of information technology?

Establishing a learning culture: help to provide information on good practice for team members whenever opportunities occur; help people to learn how to manage problems themselves rather than taking over.

Managing resources and services: identify the extra resources that might be required to provide good-quality provision; the skill mix required for delivering contraceptive care; the implications for other services and resources if staff are to add new services to their present roles.

Establishing a research and development culture: set up an automatic information-gathering service for articles about provision and management of contraceptive care on a website; conduct 'before-and-after' study of contraceptive care in the practice and PCO.

Reliable and accurate data: enter data once, consistently and correctly, and be able to retrieve it for a variety of uses and be able to compare the data with others.

Evidence-based practice and policy: find out what has worked elsewhere, and how well proven the practices are.

Confidentiality: ensure that the data is protected against unauthorised access and not passed to others without knowing the degree of confidentiality it will be given. Communicate the importance given to confidentiality so that all staff and patients are aware of the rules. Make sure that informed consent is obtained before any named data is given to others.

Health gain: the provision of good-quality contraceptive care helps to prevent unwanted pregnancy, morbidity and social exclusion.

Coherent team: everyone needs to know best practice for the provision and management of contraceptive care.

Audit and evaluation: follow the management of specific methods of contraception; learn to search and audit management and incidents in a multiplicity of ways.

Meaningful involvement of patients and the public: interactive sessions with patients and public to inform them and show ways of providing good contraceptive care; information from leaflets, computer programs and posters.

Health promotion: target health promotion with specific reminders on screen, or select specific groups for action (e.g. for cessation of smoking, screening for chlamydia).

Risk management: ensure that up-to-date records are kept on incidents in the practice; surveys of equipment; surveys of best (or poor) working practices.

Accountability and performance: monitor before and after interventions; reward and celebrate good practice and suggestions.

Core requirements: could you work out a different skill mix in your practice team to provide better provision and management of contraceptive care?

Action learning plan (include timetabled action, expected outcomes)

Who is involved? All identified staff who need to learn about the provision and management of contraceptive care with you.

Where? Identify the sites at which training and learning will take place.

Timetabled action. Start date: . . . . . .

By 3 months: preliminary data gathered and staff involved identified.
- Skills that are already present (in the practice, PCO, health authority, etc.).
- Equipment and systems that are available (yours, and those of the practice, the PCO, or outside in a training venue).
- Training that can be obtained (to match your needs).
- Training that could take place (in the practice, at other practice(s), at college or university, or at other sites such as industry, distance learning, or some other local or distant venue).
- How it could be done (individual or group; tutor-led or cascade learning).

By 6 months: review current performance.
- Are your skills being utilised in the most effective way?
- Do the building, equipment and working practices meet the specifications both for the tasks you are required to perform now and for those you anticipate doing in the immediate future?

By 7 months: identify solutions and associated learning needs.
- Arrange the necessary training.
- Make a business plan for any associated equipment needs.
- Arrange cover for yourself and any other staff who are involved to provide protected time for learning.
- Clarify who does what and when.
- Negotiate changes necessary at practice meeting(s).

By 12 months: make the changes.
- Implement the new procedures.
- Obtain feedback from other staff with regard to their impact.

- Iron out any difficulties.
- Identify any gaps in the provision.

Expected outcomes: increase in uptake of contraception; decrease in number of unwanted pregnancies; better planning of wanted pregnancies; fewer discontinuations of contraception due to inadequate information or poor management; increased screening and identification of chlamydia and other STIs in at-risk patients; better identification and management of sexual problems.

How does your personal development plan tie in with your other strategic plans? (For example, the practice's business or development plan, the local Health Improvement Programme or the Primary Care Investment Plan)

Make sure that your objectives mesh with theirs. They may have a priority for the prevention of teenage pregnancy, STIs, or the development of shared protocols for the management of sexual health matters between primary, intermediate and secondary care, into which you can feed your personal development plan.

What additional resources will you require to execute your plan and from where do you hope to obtain them?

Your entitlement to reimbursement of course fees, etc., will depend both on your contract and on the priority value that the practice or PCO puts on your development plan to meet their own needs.

Any additional equipment, alterations to the use of the building or changes in working practices will have to be decided on the same basis.

How will you evaluate your learning plan?

Look at the methods you used to identify your learning needs. How do they all fit? Can you repeat a measure that you adopted to establish your learning needs to determine how much you have learned or the extent to which your performance has improved?

How will you know when you have achieved your objectives?

You will be able to carry out the tasks you have set yourself, or you will have implemented the changes specified in your objectives list. Most of these can be audited to measure change.

How will you disseminate the learning from your plan to the rest of the practice team and patients? How will you sustain your new-found knowledge or skills?

You might let everyone know in a practice newsletter. Let the staff know what has been achieved, or what is now available, at team meetings.

Pass on your skills to other people in the team as required, and keep using your skills to provide information or better working practices. You could run an in-house training session to teach others in the practice team how to do one of the new procedures you have mastered (e.g. search and audit).

How will you handle new learning requirements as they crop up?

Keep a record as they arise, to consider later, or add them in if they are essential at this stage.

Check whether the topic you have chosen to learn is a priority and the way in which you plan to learn about it is appropriate.

> **Your topic:** *provision and management of contraceptive care*

How have you identified your learning need(s)?

(a) PCO requirement	X	(e) Appraisal need	☐
(b) Practice business plan	X	(f) New to post	☐
(c) Legal mandatory requirement (Health and Safety)	X	(g) Individual decision	X
		(h) Patient feedback	☐
(d) Job requirement	X	(i) Other	☐

Have you discussed or planned your learning needs with anyone else?

Yes X   No ☐   If so, who? *Other staff; PCO tutor and clinical governance lead.*

What are your learning need(s) and/or objective(s) in terms of the following?

> **Knowledge.** What new information do you hope to gain to help you to do this?
>
> *To learn how to implement strategies for the provision and management of contraceptive care.*
>
> **Skills.** What should you be able to do differently as a result of undertaking this learning in your development plan?
>
> *Identify best working practices; correct poor working practices; identify risky situations; identify at-risk groups and implement prevention.*
>
> **Behaviour/professional practice.** How will this impact on the way in which you then do things?
>
> *Regular reviews of services; regular reviews of standards of care for target groups.*

Details and date of desired development activity:

Within 3 months: collect sufficient information. Within 6 months: start to implement changes to working practices and management of target groups with information and interactive sessions with those patients and staff and with the wider public.

Details of any previous training and/or experience that you have in this area/dates:

Piecemeal self-instruction without structure or specific objectives.

What is your current performance in this area compared with the requirements of your job?

Need significant development in this area	☒	Need some development in this area	☐
Satisfactory in this area	☐	Do well in this area	☐

What is the level of job relevance that this area has to your role and responsibilities?

Has no relevance to job	☐	Has some relevance	☐
Relevant to job	☐	Very relevant	☒
Essential to job	☐		

Describe how the proposed education/training is relevant to your job:
Integral part of my work in the practice team.

Do you need additional support in identifying a suitable development activity?

Yes   ☒   No   ☐

What do you need?

To know when and where relevant sessions of training are being held. Help in accessing the basic information. Help with setting up staff, patient and public sessions. Help in developing services.

Describe the differences or improvements for you, your practice, PCO and/or NHS trust as a result of undertaking this activity:
I will be able to evaluate the working practices, standards of equipment and premises, standards of prevention and management, monitor performance and assess progress towards targets set by the practice team and PCO.

Assess the priority of your proposed educational/training activity:

Urgent ☐   High ☒   Medium ☐   Low ☐

Describe how the proposed activity will meet your learning needs rather than any other type of course or training on the topic:
A multidisciplinary approach is needed as the subject encompasses so many disciplines and areas of clinical and non-clinical work.

If you had a free choice, would you want to learn this?   Yes/No

If **No**, why not? (please circle all that apply)

Waste of time
I have already done it
It is not relevant to my work or career goals
Other

If **Yes**, what reasons that are most important to you? (put them in rank order):

To improve my performance	1
To increase my knowledge	2
To get promotion	

I am just interested in it
To be better than my colleagues
To do a more interesting job
To enable me to be more confident   3
Because it will help me   4
Other

Record of your learning about the provision and management of contraceptive care

You would add the date, length of time spent, etc., for each learning activity

	Activity 1 – knowledge of best practice in the provision of contraceptive services	Activity 2 – increase knowledge and skills with regard to long-acting methods of contraception	Activity 3 – setting up public involvement	Activity 4 – setting up a search and audits for monitoring best practice
In-house formal learning	Arrange for an innovator from another district to talk to the practice team and other invited professionals	Arrange for an expert to talk about long-acting methods to the practice team; draw up a resource list of provision	Health promotion staff provide a speaker to talk about how public involvement can be achieved	Set up learning sessions in the practice with the people who have skills in this area
External courses	Attend a conference on the various ways in which contraceptive services are provided in other districts	Attend a teaching community contraceptive and sexual health clinic to learn more and gain new skills	Attend a course that includes presentations on public involvement in other districts	
Informal and personal	Read articles about what others have done; discuss how the sexual health strategy can be implemented in the practice and the PCO	Discussion with practice team and PCO about how provision could be improved; practise and disseminate what has been learned	Talk to others who have done this before; involve other members of the practice team, including the health visitors and school nurses; involve schools and community resources	Informal sessions with team members; practising extracting necessary data; ensuring that data are entered in a consistent manner
Qualifications and/or experience gained	Attendance certificate	Certificate of competence in long-acting method(s); increased knowledge about provision	Experience in public participation and liaison with non-medical and paramedical sources of help	Speed and accuracy of data production and report writing

References

1 The Faculty of Family Planning and Reproductive Health Care of the Royal College of Obstetricians and Gynaecologists, 19 Cornwall Terrace, Regent's Park, London NW1 4QP.

2 Hughes L (2000) Developing primary care services for young people. *Br J Fam Plan*. **26**: 155–60.

3 Chambers R, Wakley G and Chambers S (2000) *Tackling Teenage Pregnancy: sex, culture and needs*. Radcliffe Medical Press, Oxford.

4 Donovan C, Hadley A, Jones M *et al*. (2000) *Confidentiality and Young People: a toolkit*. Royal College of General Practitioners and Brook Advisory Centre, London.

5 Maurice WL (1999) *Sexual Medicine in Primary Care*. Mosby Inc., St Louis, MO.

6 Carter Y, Moss C and Weyman A (1998) *RCGP Handbook of Sexual Health in Primary Care*. Royal College of General Practitioners, London.

7 Hannaford P and Webb A (1996) Evidence-guided prescribing of oral contraceptives. *Contraception*. **54**: 125–9.

8 Faculty of Family Planning and Reproductive Medicine (2000) Emergency contraception: recommendations for clinical practice. *Br J Fam Plan*. **26**: 93–6.

9 Bigrigg A, Evans M, Gbolade B *et al*. (1999) Depo-Provera. Position paper on clinical use, effectiveness and side effects. *Br J Fam Plan*. **25**: 69–76.

10 Guillebaud J (1999) *Contraception: your questions answered* (3e). Churchill Livingstone, London.

11 Glasier A and Gebbie A (2000) *Family Planning and Reproductive Health Care* (4e). Churchill Livingstone, London.

12 Montford H and Skrine R (1993) *Contraceptive Care: meeting individual needs*. Chapman & Hall, London.

CHAPTER 11

Draw and apply up your practice or workplace personal and professional development plan

The practice or workplace personal and professional development plan (PPDP) should cater for everyone who works in the practice. Clinical governance principles will balance the development needs of the population, the practice, the primary care organisation *and* your individual personal development plan (PDP).

You might want to start by identifying your own learning needs, combining them with those of other people and then checking them against the practice business plan. Alternatively, you could start from the other direction, by developing a practice or workplace-based personal and professional development plan from your business plan and then identifying your individual learning needs within that. Whichever direction you start from, you must ensure that you integrate your individual needs with those of your practice and the needs and directives of the NHS.

Your learning plan should complement the professional development both of other individuals and of the practice. If you are working on a project that involves change for other people as well as yourself, it is better to work together towards a common goal and co-ordinate multi-professional learning across traditional boundaries. Multiprofessional learning does not mean sitting together all learning the same information, but rather that you all learn together and individually as appropriate to your roles and responsibilities. Then all of the practice team members will understand and respect each other's contributions to provide co-ordinated patient-centred care.

If you work in a number of different roles or posts, gaps and duplication of activities should be avoided. After reflection about the boundaries between your roles, you may be able to focus your learning so that meeting your needs in one role benefits another.

Make your learning plan flexible. You may want to add something in later when circumstances suddenly change or an additional need becomes apparent – perhaps as a result of a complaint or hearing something new at a meeting.

Remember to include all those staff who work for the practice however few their hours – you cannot manage without them or they would not be there! Long-term locums (longer than six months, say), assistants, retained doctors and salaried GPs should all be included in the practice or workplace plan.

Time is one of the resources that must be considered when drawing up your action plan. Adequate resources must be in place for your learning needs, and protected time must be built in.

Template for your practice or workplace personal and professional development plan

Photocopy the following pages and complete one chart per topic.

What topic have you chosen?

Who chose it?

Justify why this topic is a priority:

(i)   *A personal or professional priority?*

(ii) *A practice priority?*

(iii) *A district priority?*

(iv) *A national priority?*

Who will be included in your practice or workplace-based personal and professional development plan?
(Anyone other than you? Doctors, nurses, employed staff, attached staff, others from outside the practice or workplace, patients?)

Who will collect the baseline information and how?

How will you identify your learning needs?
(How will you obtain this information and who will do it? Self-completion check-lists, discussion, appraisal, audit, patient feedback?)

What are the learning needs of the practice or workplace and how do they match your needs?

Is there any patient or public input to your practice or workplace development plan?

What are the aims of your practice or workplace development plan arising from the preliminary data-gathering exercise?

How might you integrate the 14 components of clinical govern-ance into your practice or workplace personal and professional development plan focusing on the topic of . . . . ?

Establishing a learning culture:

Managing resources and services:

Establishing a research and development culture:

Reliable and accurate data:

Evidence-based practice and policy:

Confidentiality:

Health gain:

Coherent team:

Audit and evaluation:

Meaningful involvement of patients and the public:

Health promotion:

Risk management:

Accountability and performance:

Core requirements:

Action learning plan (include timetabled action and expected outcomes)

How does your practice or workplace development plan tie in with your other strategic plans?
(For example, the practice's business or development plan, the local Health Improvement Programme, the Primary Care Investment Plan or the Trust Development Plan)

What additional resources will you require to execute your plan and from where do you hope to obtain them?
(Will you have to pay any course fees? Will you be able to organise any protected time for learning in working hours?)

How will you evaluate your practice or workplace personal and professional development plan?

How will you know when you have achieved your objectives?
(How will you measure success?)

**How will you disseminate the learning from your plan to the rest
of the team and patients? How will you sustain your new-found
knowledge or skills?**

How will you handle new learning requirements as they crop up?

Record of your learning

Write in the topic, date, time spent and type of learning

	Activity 1	Activity 2	Activity 3	Activity 4
In-house formal learning				
External courses				
Informal and personal				
Qualifications and/or experience gained				

Worked example

Practice personal and professional development plan focusing on providing a specialist sexual health service for the primary care organisation (PCO)

Who chose the topic?

Many of the practice team realise that improving the care of patients with sexual health needs is of increasing importance after the preliminary learning needs assessment. The district or PCO is undertaking a strategic review of provision of services for meeting sexual health needs following the introduction of a local sexual health strategy. Inconsistent management and patchy provision for at-risk groups have been revealed so far.

Justify why this topic is a priority?

(i) *A practice and professional priority?* Good risk management is an essential part of care at a clinical level for individuals with sexual health needs. Risk management is also important from an organisational perspective for identifying those at risk, preventing unwanted pregnancies and STIs, and reducing abortions and morbidity. Therefore investing time and effort in improving the care of those with sexual health needs should produce tangible and significant health gains for individual patients.

(ii) *A district priority?* Several other districts have already set up schemes to improve the provision for sexual health needs. They have local initiatives to co-ordinate the management of those with sexual health needs and to provide more 'seamless' care across the primary/secondary care interface (e.g. by amalgamating genitourinary medicine (GUM) and contraceptive care, and providing sexual problem management by GPs and nurses with special interest and skills).

(iii) *A national priority?* The cost of the effects of not meeting sexual health needs is high. Effective prevention is cost-effective to the NHS, through avoiding unwanted pregnancies and reducing morbidity, and minimising the effects of poor sexual health on physical and psychosocial functioning. The new national sexual health strategy, drawn up after extensive consultation, will indicate what services should be developed to meet sexual health needs more effectively.

Who will be included in your practice or workplace-based personal and professional development plan?

You might include the following:

- patients with sexual health needs, and their partners
- GPs
- practice nurses
- school nurses
- health visitors
- district nurses
- health education staff
- community pharmacists
- practice manager
- reception staff
- youth workers
- representatives from education and social services
- representatives from community contraceptive care, GUM, urology and gynaecology and physiotherapy departments.

Who will collect the baseline information and how?

A receptionist/computer operator could conduct an electronic search in your practice to identify individuals with sexual health needs, and the associated risk factors, if appropriately coded. Otherwise it will be laborious to set up an at-risk register from discharge letters from hospital, paper records, repeat prescriptions, recall, etc. A needs assessment of your area might be used by the PCO to establish what services are needed and where. Once you know who the groups are that you want to target, you can audit their care and see what you need to learn.

The local public health department at your health authority should be able to supply data about pregnancy rates, STI rates, sexual difficulties, and morbidity and mortality rates in your district. They may also have national data on file about the average numbers per 1000 population who might be expected to have sexual health needs, categorised by age, gender and ethnic group, or you can obtain this information from your local medical library.

The local hospital trust could give you routine and acute data about referrals and admissions of those with sexual health problems or unwanted pregnancies. The hospital audit department may have undertaken work on teenage pregnancy rates, abortion care, or treatment of chlamydia, and might give you a breakdown of results identifying your patient or PCO populations.

Where are you now? (Baseline)

- Establish how many people with sexual health needs you might be catering for. Set up criteria for identifying at-risk groups, and list them by age groups.
- Compare your practice guidelines for managing each sexual health need with a guideline cited in the literature as 'best practice' or a recommended district protocol. If you do not have a practice protocol, write one or adopt someone else's (*see* the individual chapters for details).
- Find out where else your patients go to obtain contraceptive services, and whether this is more convenient or acceptable for them.
- Focus on the prevention of avoidable risks – such as looking at the number who become pregnant after receiving contraceptive advice, who might have benefited from other methods of contraception, who need second abortions, who develop pelvic infections or reinfection with chlamydia after treatment, etc.
- Assess the quantity and quality of literature that is available for patients and their partners in your practice.
- Review the extent of education or training that the clinical staff have received about meeting sexual health needs.
- Undertake an analysis of the strengths, weaknesses, opportunities and threats (SWOT) of your practice team in managing and preventing sexual health needs.

What information will you obtain about individual learning wishes and needs?

You might review practice protocols and baseline information with as many staff as possible at discussion groups and find out whether they feel competent as individuals to carry out their roles and responsibilities, or if they wish to realign their duties. They might comment on how well others are fulfilling their responsibilities and suggest improvements to the systems or procedures that have educational and resource consequences – training sessions, new equipment, and especially the effects on other parts of the practice organisation of introducing new services.

A significant event audit (e.g. that of a person who presents with an unwanted pregnancy after receiving contraceptive advice, or with pelvic inflammatory disease, or who has numerous unnecessary investigations for what turns out to be a sexual problem).

What are the learning needs of the practice and how do they match the needs of individuals?

Responding to queries from the PCO about the practice's management of sexual health needs might reveal inadequacies in your baseline knowledge of what services you are providing, how they are utilised or what you are achieving. This might create the opportunity to review how individuals contribute to the overall care provided – include the employed and attached staff as well as individuals such as the local community pharmacist or local youth worker. Once you are sure of everyone's roles and responsibilities and your vision for the care that you intend to provide, you can re-assess individuals' learning needs in a co-ordinated plan to match the service you will provide.

Compare your own figures for the number of individuals with sexual health needs with those you would expect in a practice population of the same size and demographic make-up. Decide whether you need to be more pro-active in identifying at-risk groups or new cases of sexual health needs, and address lack of knowledge or skills, and uncaring attitudes or inadequate systems.

Compare the prescribing patterns of the GPs in your practice with those in other practices. Look for differences and inconsistencies that may indicate learning needs.

A patient complaint may reveal learning needs for individuals or the practice organisation (e.g. the case of a patient who did not have adequate swabs taken to investigate her complaint of bleeding after intercourse, and who went on to develop a pelvic infection and loss of fertility).

Compare your practice guidelines for the management of sexual health needs with other recommended guidelines in order to reveal learning needs.

The practice nurse or health visitor might have nominated sexual health problems as a topic they wished to learn more about at their annual job appraisal. If no one else in the practice has expert knowledge or skills in the management of sexual health problems, then it will be well worth the practice facilitating the nurse to attend an in-depth course.

The practice manager may intend to visit other areas to find out how others manage their services for the provision of a sexual health service. This focus might justify additional time spent on practice or clinic visiting.

Is there any patient or public input to your practice or workplace development plan?

Ask the patient who made a complaint or comment to help you to devise better systems in the practice or to write an account of their experiences that can be used for an in-house training session.

You might ask the health adviser from the GUM clinic or an expert who has set up a service elsewhere to attend an informal training session – in particular dealing with educating and informing patients more effectively, and motivating patients with regard to prevention of risks and side-effects of treatment.

An open forum on sexual health needs can be held for all those staff who will be involved to provide an opportunity for everyone to mix and exchange ideas. Informal conversations during the event should reveal learning needs and ideas for improvements.

What are the aims of your practice or workplace personal and professional development plan arising from the preliminary data-gathering exercise?

After collecting baseline data and undertaking a preliminary learning needs assessment, you might design a practice personal and professional development plan that has the grand overarching aim of developing a learning programme for all members of the practice team, attached staff and individuals, to enable them to provide an effective specialist sexual health service for the PCO within the available resources.

Alternatively, you might concentrate on developing particular key individuals (e.g. a GP or practice nurse and specific receptionist with lead responsibility for the clinical management or practice organisation for meeting sexual health needs). They could then cascade their learning in-house to others in the practice team.

Yet another option would be to focus on specific aspects of the effective management of sexual health needs (e.g. what swabs need to be taken, how to manage erectile dysfunction, or how to motivate people to use contraception consistently).

Another aim would be to develop a learning programme for all members of the wider primary healthcare team, to increase their knowledge and skills in educating and informing patients and their partners about the prevention of sexual health problems. This might include learning how to motivate patients to understand recommended management practices, avoid risks and complications, complete treatment, make lifestyle changes or use contraception consistently.

How might you integrate the 14 components of clinical governance into your practice personal and professional development plan focusing on providing a specialist sexual health service for the PCO?

Establishing a learning culture: a multidisciplinary team might update their learning about the risk factors for sexual health problems. The practice manager could learn about setting up services to meet sexual health needs. The nurses and GPs could gain more knowledge and skills to meet sexual health needs.

Managing resources and services: promote close working relationships and teamwork between the practice staff, and others involved in the wider community, such as school nurses, youth workers, social services and education. Provide new services to fill the gaps and reduce duplication of effort. Advertise services that are available to all members of the population in the area of one PCO.

Establishing a research and development culture: encourage practice team members to critically appraise published papers describing new findings with regard to sexual health needs, in order to check whether the results described are applicable to their population.

Reliable and accurate data: keep good records to enable evaluation of the service provided and establish how it can be monitored and improved.

Evidence-based practice and policy: the guidelines for people with various sexual health needs should be based on the best evidence for the population and local circumstances.

Confidentiality: there should be water-tight systems in place to prevent any information about a patient having sexual health needs or risk factors for sexual health problems being released without their consent. Any issues of confidentiality should be clarified before information about individuals is passed to others.

Health gain: prevention and treatment of STIs, prevention of unwanted pregnancy, or help with sexual problems; improvement of health and well-being.

Coherent team: all members of the practice team should understand each other's roles and responsibilities in providing care.

Audit and evaluation: a significant event audit (e.g. of a person with risk factors having a pelvic infection or abortion) should indicate areas where further training is required, or where practice services and teamwork need to be improved.

Meaningful involvement of patients and the public: you might hold a public session in the surgery, or elsewhere, demonstrating strategies for meeting sexual health needs. An assessment questionnaire for identifying sexual health needs might identify areas that are not being met already. A focus group of patients with sexual health needs might reveal shortcomings in staff knowledge and attitudes, or malfunctioning practice systems, or lack of appropriate services.

Health promotion: target patients at risk of sexual health problems with advice about their lifestyle – not by means of negative messages, but as part of an attempt to increase their ability to enjoy their sexuality in a healthy way.

Risk management: identification and control of risks is part of the purpose of providing a specialist sexual health service for the PCO, to reduce the likelihood and extent of infertility and infection, unwanted pregnancies, physical or psychological disability associated with sexual problems, dependence or premature death.

Accountability and performance: demonstrate that the advice and treatment which staff are providing to people with sexual health needs are in line with best practice.

Core requirements: staff should be competent in and trained for their roles and responsibilities. Think about skill mix and other appropriately trained professionals (e.g. Relate counsellors or GUM health advisers).

Action learning plan (include timetabled action and expected outcomes)

Who is involved?/What is the setting? Staff as set out previously (specify names and posts).

Timetabled action. Start date: . . . . .

By 3 months: preliminary data gathering and collation of baseline of providers of sexual health services.

- Is there guidance on providing a specialist sexual health service for the PCO?
- Numbers of staff; map expertise; list other providers of sexual health services.
- Referral patterns for routine advice and monitoring of sexual health needs; referrals to secondary care for termination of pregnancy, infections, complications or complex problems.
- Information about the characteristics of those recorded as having sexual health needs (age groups, ethnic origins).
- Any relevant local and national priorities, and any additional associated resources for which you might apply.
- Staff discussion to report problems that limit individuals of different age groups, etc. with sexual health needs accessing services, the problems, and their views and suggestions.

By 4 months: review current performance.
- Practice manager reviews operation of services and closeness of working relationships with those in other organisations and sectors who have an interest in or responsibility for the provision of a specialist sexual health service for the PCO.
- Clinical leads (e.g. GP, nurse) review the extent of the knowledge, skills and attitudes of the practice team with regard to the provision of a specialist sexual health service for the PCO.
- Audit actual performance vs. pre-agreed criteria (e.g. with regard to referrals, education given to those with risk factors for or established sexual health needs and investigations, monitoring and compliance).
- Compare actual performance with one or more of the 14 components of clinical governance (e.g. health promotion would be very relevant).

By 6 months: identify solutions and associated training needs.
- Set up new systems for access to services appropriate to the provision of a specialist sexual health service for the PCO.
- Give the practice team in-house training in important aspects of the provision of a specialist sexual health service for the PCO.
- Revise the guidelines. Address identified gaps in care, having undertaken searches for other evidence-based guidelines. Agree on roles and responsibilities as a team for delivering care and services according to protocol; certain staff attend external courses. Practice or school nurse, GP, pharmacist, GUM specialists, family planning instructing doctors and nurses provide some in-house training to other GPs and nurses, the community pharmacist or others from outside organisations with whom the practice is liaising about the issue.

By 12 months: make changes.
- Clinicians adhere to the practice protocol, as shown by repeat audits and patient feedback.
- Change service times and locations to make them more appropriate for those with sexual health needs of various age ranges, disabilities and ethnic groups, having organised training to anticipate new requirements (e.g. train youth workers to give the same advice as other members of the primary care team).

Expected outcomes: more effective provision of a specialist sexual health service for the PCO; better patient compliance with treatment, and good lifestyle habits; fewer unwanted pregnancies and infections; better management of sexual problems.

How does your practice or workplace personal and professional development plan tie in with your other strategic plans?

The practice's business plan and the PCO's Primary Care Investment Plan might both prioritise the achievement of more effective provision for a specialist sexual health service for the PCO. The practice personal and professional development plan that focuses on providing a specialist sexual health service for the PCO would complement those strategic plans.

What additional resources will you require to execute your plan and from where do you hope to obtain them?

The practice might pay for the course fees of any member of staff undertaking training that fulfils a priority need of the practice.

You may be able to justify an application for additional resources to your PCO or health authority or local NHS trust with your preliminary learning and health needs assessments, tapping into the district or national strategic priorities. You should point out that this expenditure would be balanced by savings from the better management of sexual health needs.

If a member of staff is undertaking the training on behalf of the practice, you should try to arrange for the training to be undertaken in paid time. Any learning that is cascaded to other members of the practice team as part of the practice personal and professional development plan should also be undertaken in paid time and during working hours whenever possible.

How will you evaluate your practice or workplace personal and professional development plan?

You should be able to select methods of evaluation from the range of methods that you use for assessing learning needs. The most appropriate methods will depend on the specific aims that you set for your development plan. For example, if your main aim is to prevent sexual health problems in individuals with risky lifestyles, you might evaluate this by monitoring the number of people who develop STIs and unwanted pregnancies. However, if your aim is to improve the levels and appropriateness of education and information for people with unmet sexual health needs, you might want to ask the patients themselves – by a simple test of knowledge, focus group discussion of experiences, monitoring changes in patient behaviour, etc.

The practice manager and clinical lead for providing a specialist sexual health service for the PCO (e.g. a GP or practice nurse) might plan the evaluation together and delegate the collection of data to a receptionist.

How will you know when you have achieved your objectives?

Usually this will be by comparing the outcomes of your programme with baseline data. However, it might also be determined by looking at patients' compliance with recommended practice, or the lifestyle changes that they have achieved.

How will you disseminate the learning from your plan to the rest of the practice team and patients? How will you sustain your new-found knowledge and skills?

You might write about it in a practice newsletter. Let all the staff know at practice meetings what progress has been made. You might want to describe your success at a PCO meeting, or apply for an award for best practice from one of the national GP newspapers. Pass on your skills and knowledge to others as required, and review your protocol at set intervals in order to incorporate new information.

How will you handle new learning requirements as they crop up?

The practice manager might run audits at intervals and feed the results back to a practice meeting. This might take place half-way through the time period of the development plan when there is time to revise the activities.

Record of practice team learning about the provision of a specialist sexual health service for the PCO

You would add the date, length of time spent, etc., for each learning activity

	Activity 1 – revise practice guidelines and protocols	*Activity 2 – update patient education*	*Activity 3 – management of sexual health problems*	*Activity 4 – managing STIs and related disorders*
In-house formal learning	Practice team discussion of the roles and responsibilities of various members to fulfil protocols – including school nurses, youth workers and others	The health adviser from the GUM clinic runs an interactive session about educating people with sexual health risks, with GPs, nurses and other interested individuals	GP and nurse share ideas with the rest of the practice team during practice discussion of sexual health problems and protocols (*see* Activity 1)	Hospital specialist input to practice team discussion when changes to practice protocols are reviewed, with any changes to medication for established STIs
External courses	GP/nurse lead attends two-day continuing education course on sexual health needs at regional centre		GP and/or practice nurse attends courses on the management of sexual health problems	Practice nurse and GP attend course on management of STIs
Informal and personal	Practice nurse and GP search for examples of best practice on Medline at home. Practice manager telephones other practices and clinics to ask for examples of protocols	Health visitor brings in all of the available literature and audio-visual aids on sexual health needs. Team sorts them according to criteria agreed for evaluation of patient information	GP/practice nurse picks up tips from other course members and discusses the management of sexual health problems with other members of staff as they occur	Practice team members all learn from talking to the GP and practice nurse about the day-to-day investigation and treatment of STIs and related disorders
Qualifications and/or experience gained	GP/nurse lead receives accreditation that can be added to their learning portfolio	Reflective learning	Certificate or diploma in sexual health problem management; reflective learning from patient management	Certificate of attendance at course; reflective learning from patient management

Sources of help

Useful websites

Caution: websites often change or disappear.

On guidelines

Agency for Health Care Policy and Research (AHCPR)	http://www.guideline.gov
Bandolier	http://ebandolier.com
Canadian Medical Association	http://www.cma.ca/cpgs/
Cochrane Collaboration	http://www.cochrane.org
*e*Guidelines	http://www.eguidelines.co.uk
General Medical Council	http://www.gmc-uk.org
Guideline Appraisal Project	http://www.cche.net/principles/content_all.asp
Guideline Project	http://www.jr2.ox.ac.uk
HoN (Health on the Net)	http://www.hon.ch
Medline	http://www.omni.ac.uk/medline
New Zealand Guidelines Group	http://www.nzgg.org.nz/index.htm
NLM Health Services/Technology Assessment	http://www.nlm.nih.gov
North of England Evidence-Based Guidelines	http://www.ncl.ac.uk/~ncenthsr/publicn/guide/guide.htm
OMNI (Organising Medical Networked Information)	http://www.omni.ac.uk
PRODIGY	http://www.prodigy.nhs.uk
Scottish Intercollegiate Guidelines Network (SIGN)	http://www.sign.ac.uk
St George's Health Care Evaluation Unit	http://www.sghms.ac.uk/depts/phs/hceu/nhsguide.htm
UK Health Centre	http://www.healthcentre.org.uk/hc/library/guidelines.htm
WISDOM Centre	http://www.wisdomnet.co.uk

On sexual health matters

British Association for Sexual and Relationship Therapy	http://www.basrt.org.uk
British Medical Journal	http://www.bmj.com
British Sexual Health Information Service	http://www.shastd.org.uk
Elisa testing	http://www.hometest.co.uk/ Endomysial-antibodies.html
Erectile dysfunction evidence: (there are also thousands of other sites)	http://jr2.ox.ac.uk
Faculty of Family Planning and Reproductive Health Care	http://www.ffprhc.org.uk
Family Planning Association	http://www.fpa.org.uk
Genitourinary Medicine guidelines	http://www.agum.org.uk
Institute of Psychosexual Medicine	http://www.ipm.org.uk
Lancet	http://www.thelancet.com
National AIDS Manual	http://www.aidsmap.com
National AIDS Trust	http://www.nat.org.uk
National Electronic Library for Health	http://www.nelh.nhs.uk
Public Health Laboratory Service	http://phls.co.uk
The pill and cancer (Medicines Control Agency)	http://www.ukonline.gov.uk
Terence Higgins Trust (AIDS site)	http://www.tht.org.uk

Index